50% OFF
Online NCLEX-RN Prep Course!

Dear Customer,

Thank you for your purchase of this NCLEX-RN Study Guide. Included with your purchase is **discounted access to our online NCLEX-RN Prep Course.** Many courses cost hundreds of dollars and don't deliver enough value. Our course provides the best NCLEX-RN prep material, and with discounted access, **you only pay half price.**

We have structured our online course to perfectly complement your printed study guide. The NCLEX-RN Prep Course contains **in-depth lessons** that cover all the most important topics, **110+ video reviews** that explain difficult concepts, over **1,600 practice questions** to ensure you feel prepared, and over **1,000 digital flashcards,** so you can fit some studying in while you're on the go.

Online NCLEX-RN Prep Course

Topics Covered:

- Management of Care
  - o Case Management
  - o Collaborative Care Management
  - o Ethical Practices
- Safety and Infection Control
  - o Accident, Error, and Injury Prevention
  - o Emergency Response
  - o Infectious Diseases and Infection Control
- Health Promotion and Maintenance
  - o Developmental Stages and Transitions
  - o Disease Prevention
  - o Health Screening
- And More!

Course Features:

- NCLEX-RN Study Guide
  - o Get content that complements our best-selling study guide.
- 12 Full-Length Practice Tests
  - o With over 1,600 practice questions, you can test yourself again and again.
- Mobile Friendly
  - o If you need to study on the go, the course is easily accessible from your mobile device.
- NCLEX-RN Flashcards
  - o Our course includes a flashcard mode consisting of over 1,000 content cards to help you study.

To lock in your discounted access, visit mometrix.com/university/nclex-rn or simply scan this QR code with your smartphone. At the checkout page, enter the discount code: **nclex50off**

If you have any questions or concerns, please contact us at support@mometrix.com.

Sincerely,

M✓metrix
TEST PREPARATION

SCAN HERE

NCLEX-RN® Practice Questions

NCLEX® Practice Tests & Exam Review for
the National Council Licensure Examination
for Registered Nurses

Mometrix
TEST PREPARATION

Written and edited by the Mometrix Nursing Certification Test Team

Mometrix offers volume discount pricing to institutions. For more information or a price quote, please contact our sales department at sales@mometrix.com or 888-248-1219.

Paperback
ISBN 13: 978-1-61403-603-6
ISBN 10: 1-61403-603-9

Ebook
ISBN 13: 978-1-62733-509-6
ISBN 10: 1-62733-509-9

Hardback
ISBN 13: 978-1-5167-0811-6
ISBN 10: 1-5167-0811-3

DEAR FUTURE EXAM SUCCESS STORY

First of all, **THANK YOU** for purchasing Mometrix study materials!

Second, congratulations! You are one of the few determined test-takers who are committed to doing whatever it takes to excel on your exam. **You have come to the right place.** We developed these study materials with one goal in mind: to deliver you the information you need in a format that's concise and easy to use.

In addition to optimizing your guide for the content of the test, we've outlined our recommended steps for breaking down the preparation process into small, attainable goals so you can make sure you stay on track.

We've also analyzed the entire test-taking process, identifying the most common pitfalls and showing how you can overcome them and be ready for any curveball the test throws you.

Standardized testing is one of the biggest obstacles on your road to success, which only increases the importance of doing well in the high-pressure, high-stakes environment of test day. Your results on this test could have a significant impact on your future, and this guide provides the information and practical advice to help you achieve your full potential on test day.

Your success is our success

We would love to hear from you! If you would like to share the story of your exam success or if you have any questions or comments in regard to our products, please contact us at **800-673-8175** or **support@mometrix.com**.

Thanks again for your business and we wish you continued success!

Sincerely,
The Mometrix Test Preparation Team

TABLE OF CONTENTS

Practice Test #1

Case Study 1

A 23-year-old female is brought into the emergency department by her mother.

Nurses' Notes

1600: A 23-year-old female client arrives at the emergency department with her mother. The client appears tearful and withdrawn, and she is clutching her abdomen. Her mother reports receiving a concerning call from her daughter approximately 1 hour prior to their arrival, and, when she went to check on her, she found that the client had taken a handful of acetaminophen. The client admits to taking approximately fifteen 325 mg acetaminophen tablets at approximately 1300 with the intent to end her life. The client states that she got into an argument with her significant other earlier in the day. The client is now complaining of mild abdominal pain and nausea. She has a history of depression, has been taking sertraline (Zoloft), and had a previous suicide attempt approximately 1 year ago. The client is placed on the cardiac monitor, IV access is established, labs are drawn, and a set of vitals is obtained. The client agrees to a safety contract, stating she will notify staff if she feels that she will harm herself while in the hospital.

Vital Signs

	1600
Temp	98.5 °F temporal
HR	102
BP	110/72
RR	22
Pulse oximetry	95% on room air

Physical Assessment

Body System	**1600**
Neurological	The client is alert and oriented ×4.
Psychological	The client is withdrawn and tearful, and she appears somewhat disheveled. The client's mother appears to be supportive.
Cardiovascular	The client's heart rhythm is sinus tachycardia; pulses are strong and regular.
Integumentary	Old scars are noted with superficial laceration scars to the wrists.
Gastrointestinal (GI)	Mild abdominal cramping and nausea. Bowel sounds are active. The client's abdomen is nontender.

1

LABORATORY RESULTS

Laboratory Test and Reference Range	1600
Hemoglobin (Hgb) Female: 12–15 g/dL	14
White blood cell (WBC) count Adult/child >2 years: 5,000–10,000/mm³	8,500
Acetaminophen <20 mcg/mL	30
ALT Female: 7–30 units/L	25
AST Female: 9–32 units/L	30
Blood ethanol Adult: <10 mg/dL	185

1. From the following list, select the assessment findings that require <u>immediate</u> follow-up. (Select all that apply)

1. Heart rate
2. Ingested acetaminophen dosage
3. Client history
4. ALT/AST
5. Serum acetaminophen
6. Blood ethanol
7. Respiratory rate

2. If left untreated, the client is at the highest risk of developing _____.

1. acute kidney failure
2. cirrhosis
3. gastrointestinal (GI) bleed
4. acute liver failure

3. The nurse receives the following orders. Highlight all orders from the following list that the nurse should consider a <u>priority</u>.

- Place the client on a mental health hold.
- Administer IV ondansetron.
- Obtain urinary toxicology.
- Administer IV acetylcysteine.
- Obtain a bedside urine pregnancy test.

4. For the following list of potential nursing interventions, specify whether each one is indicated or not indicated.

Potential Nursing Interventions	Indicated	Not Indicated
Request an order for repeat labs in 4 hours.	○	○
Place the client on seizure precautions.	○	○
Contact the local poison control center.	○	○
Notify the mental health team and charge nurse that the client is suicidal.	○	○
Remove cardiac monitoring from the room.	○	○
Ask the client's visitor to leave.	○	○

NURSES' NOTES

1630: The client's belongings are placed in a secure place. A sitter is at the bedside to ensure client safety. The physician notifies the client that she is on a mental health hold, and the client is given a list of her rights. The nurse administers IV acetylcysteine and IV ondansetron and contacts the local poison control center for further monitoring instructions. The client's urine toxicology came back negative for any other substances, and the client's urine pregnancy testing was also negative.

NURSES' NOTES

2000: Repeat labs are drawn, and repeat vital sign measurements are obtained. The client reports that her nausea has subsided and she appears calm, requesting a sandwich box. The client's mother leaves the bedside to get food, informing the client that she will return. The sitter remains present.

VITAL SIGNS

	1600	2000
Temp	98.5 °F temporal	97.7 °F temporal
HR	102	95
BP	110/72	115/85
RR	22	20
Pulse oximetry	95% on room air	96% on room air

LABORATORY RESULTS

Laboratory Test and Reference Range	1600	2000
Acetaminophen <20 mcg/mL	30	22
ALT Female: 7–30 units/L	25	31
AST Female: 9–32 units/L	30	35
Blood ethanol Adult: <10 mg/dL	185	125

5. For the following list of assessment findings, specify whether each one indicates that the client's condition has improved, is unchanged, or has worsened.

Assessment Findings	Improved	Unchanged	Worsened
GI symptoms	○	○	○
Liver function	○	○	○
Blood pressure, 115/85	○	○	○
Serum acetaminophen	○	○	○

6. The client is being prepared for hospital admission. Of the following statements, which indicate(s) that the client demonstrates understanding of plan of care? (Select all that apply)

1. "Because I'm being admitted, I will have no rights until I am discharged."
2. "You will be monitoring my liver function while I'm in the hospital."
3. "Once I'm medically cleared, the mental health team will come talk to me."
4. "You're going to put me in a padded room like a crazy person."
5. "I may be admitted to a mental health facility."

Case Study 2

The client is a 71-year-old male with a recent cancer diagnosis who has received four cycles of chemotherapy. He presents in the clinic today for a visit with his oncologist prior to starting cycle five of chemotherapy treatment. The client has labs drawn prior to his appointment, although the results are not available when the nurse evaluates the patient.

NURSES' NOTES

1045: Upon entering the room, the client appears pale, but well, much like previous visits. He reports being tired, but he is able to carry out his normal activities of daily living (ADLs) independently. When questioned about any new or worsened symptoms, the client reports a rash on his legs that developed 2 days ago but denies itching at the site. Upon visual inspection, the nurse finds a flat, pinpoint, reddish-purple rash on the client's bilateral lower extremities. The client also reports the continued presence of a metallic taste in his mouth and numbness and tingling of his hands and feet that has not worsened. The nurse observes a new bruise to the client's left arm that is approximately the size of a quarter. The client denies knowing the origin of this bruise.

VITAL SIGNS

	1045
Temp	98.7 °F axillary
HR	75
BP	110/76
RR	18
Pulse oximetry	98% on room air

1. From the following list, select the assessment findings that require <u>immediate</u> follow-up. (Select all that apply)

1. Metallic taste in the mouth
2. Reddish-purple rash
3. Pallor
4. Fatigue
5. Numbness and tingling of the hands and feet
6. Blood pressure 110/76
7. Bruising

2. Based on the assessment and history for this client, the nurse knows that these new findings are <u>most likely</u> indicative of _____.

1. thrombocytopenia
2. neutropenia
3. anemia
4. cachexia

CBC LABORATORY RESULTS

The nurse reviews the laboratory results that were drawn at 1030.

	1030
WBC	3.7 (L) k/µL
RBC	3.25 (L) mil/ µL
Hemoglobin	10 (L) g/dL
Hematocrit	25 (L) %
MCV	85 µm³
MCH	27 pg
MCHC	32 g/dL
RDW	18.9 (H) %
Platelet	19 (L) k/µL
MPV	8 fL

3. After review of the client's laboratory results, which value does the nurse find best correlates with her 1045 assessment findings?

1. WBC 3,700/µL
2. RBC 3.25 mil/µL
3. Hemoglobin 10 g/dL
4. Platelets 19,000/µL

4. For the following list of potential medical interventions, specify whether each one is indicated or not indicated.

Potential Medical Interventions	Indicated	Not Indicated
Arrange for a repeat CBC and nurse visit in 24 hours.	○	○
Administer IV antiemetics.	○	○
Administer IV platelets.	○	○
Administer subcutaneous heparin.	○	○
Hold cycle five of chemotherapy.	○	○

5. After completing the appropriate medical interventions, the nurse educates the client on thrombocytopenia precautions. Highlight the appropriate nursing recommendations from the list below.

- Avoid crowded places.
- Use a soft-bristled toothbrush.
- Use an electric razor.
- Take breaks between ADLs.
- Go to the emergency department (ED) if experiencing a nosebleed that will not stop.
- Take ibuprofen or naproxen for a headache.

6. For the following list of assessment findings, specify whether each one indicates that the client's condition has improved, is unchanged, or has worsened.

Assessment Findings	Improved	Unchanged	Worsened
Spontaneously bleeding gums	○	○	○
Light rash on the bilateral feet	○	○	○
Eraser tip-sized black spot on the tongue	○	○	○
Sudden sharp headache	○	○	○
Platelet count 20,000/μL	○	○	○

Case Study 3

The nurse is caring for a 58-year-old male on the cardiac unit.

<u>NURSES' NOTES</u>

Day 1, 0800: The client arrived on the unit after an episode of syncope at home that lasted 2 minutes. The client is now alert and oriented to person, place, time, and situation. Lung sounds are clear, and pulses are strong in all extremities. Bowel sounds are hypoactive in all four quadrants. Skin is pale and dry. He denies any dizziness, light-headedness, or pain. The client has a history of hypercholesteremia, hypertension, gout, and a non-ST-elevation myocardial infarction (MI) 2 years ago. The client is a smoker with a 30 pack-year history. A telemetry monitor is applied that indicates normal sinus rhythm.

Day 1, 1215: The client called the nurse to the room and reported epigastric pain that radiates to his shoulder, with nausea and difficulty breathing. The client was restless and unable to lie still in bed. His heart rhythm is regular, but the rate is elevated. Radial and pedal pulses are weak, graded 1+. Lung sounds are clear.

<u>VITAL SIGNS</u>

	0800	1215
Temp	98.5 °F axillary	98.3 °F axillary
HR	89	120
BP	132/88	80/49
RR	18	30
Pulse oximetry	92%	87%

1. The nurse reviews the assessment data and vital signs. From the following list, select the assessment findings that require <u>immediate</u> follow-up. (Select all that apply)

1. Heart rate, 120
2. Blood pressure, 80/49
3. Lung sounds
4. Bowel sounds
5. Respirations, 30
6. Diaphoresis
7. Epigastric pain

2. For the list of client findings below, specify for each whether it is consistent with the disease processes of myocardial infarction (MI), systemic inflammatory response syndrome (SIRS), or cardiogenic shock. Select all supported disease processes for each finding.

Client Findings	MI	SIRS	Cardiogenic Shock
Epigastric pain	☐	☐	☐
Diaphoresis	☐	☐	☐
Restlessness	☐	☐	☐
Nausea	☐	☐	☐
Heart rate, 120	☐	☐	☐

NURSES' NOTES

Day 1, 1225: The primary physician was notified of the client's condition and arrived at the client's bedside. Electrocardiogram completed and showed tachycardia with ST segment elevation. The client was diagnosed with an acute MI per the physician. A plan was made for a stat cardiac catheterization.

3. The nurse should recognize that the client is at the most <u>immediate</u> risk of developing _____.

1. a pneumothorax
2. cardiac arrest
3. congestive heart failure

NURSES' NOTES

Day 1, 1230: The client is no longer responding to questions or physical touch. The pulse is not palpable to the femoral or carotid arteries. The telemetry monitor shows the following:

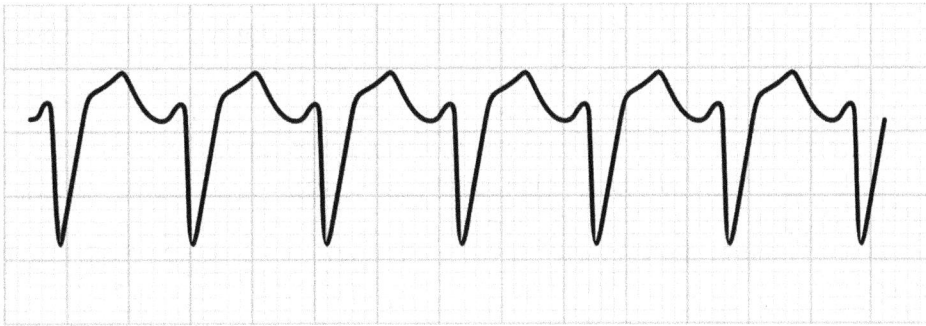

4. For the following list of potential interventions, specify whether each is indicated or not indicated.

Potential Nursing Interventions	Indicated	Not Indicated
Apply automatic external defibrillator pads, one to the upper right side of the chest and one to the lower left lateral side of the chest.	○	○
Administer a sublingual nitroglycerin 0.3 mg tablet per the facility's cardiac arrest protocol.	○	○
Apply a nonrebreather oxygen mask at 10 L/min.	○	○
Activate a code blue.	○	○
Begin chest compressions at 120 beats per minute.	○	○
Place the client in the semi-Fowler's position.	○	○

<u>NURSES' NOTES</u>

Day 1, 1235 (summary of code event): A code blue was activated, and the code team arrived. Chest compressions and rescue breaths were delivered via bag valve mask. Automatic external defibrillator pads were applied. A shock of 200 joules was delivered to the client. The cardiac monitor now shows the following rhythm. No femoral or carotid pulse is palpable.

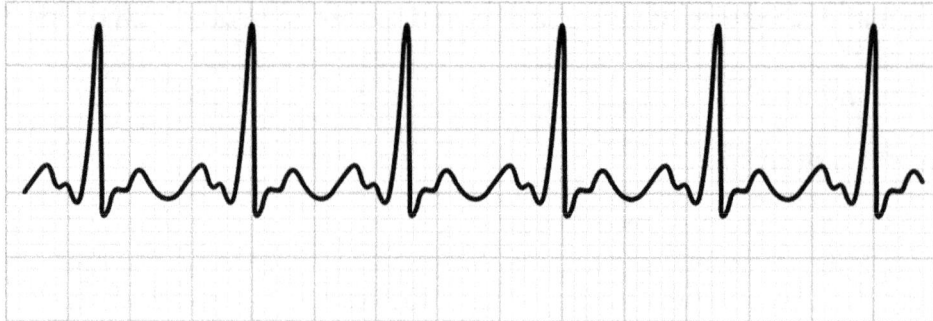

5. Highlight the orders from the following list that the nurse should anticipate based on the client's current status.

- Administer another shock of 200 joules to the client.
- Continue chest compressions at a rate of 120 times per minute.
- Stop the code because the heartbeat has returned to normal.
- Prepare a syringe of 1 mg IV epinephrine.
- Draw blood for laboratory tests: complete blood count, complete metabolic panel, arterial blood gas.

<u>NURSES' NOTES</u>

Day 3, 0800: The client is day 4 status post-MI and subsequent cardiac arrest. Pulse was reestablished following a code blue, and stat cardiac catheterization was performed with stent placement to the left anterior descending artery. The client has transferred back to the cardiac unit from the intensive care unit. Ongoing education has been provided to him in preparation for his eventual discharge.

6. Which of the following statements from the client indicates that he understands the education provided by the nurse? (Select all that apply)

1. "I will take clopidogrel daily for the next year."
2. "I will refrain from exercise for the next 2 months."
3. "I will stop taking atorvastatin."
4. "I will wait 6 months before returning to smoking again."
5. "I will follow up with the dietitian as soon as possible."

Standalone Questions

1. A client has a large pressure injury on the coccygeal area. The pressure injury is draining large amounts of seropurulent discharge. Which of the following is the most appropriate choice for dressing material?

1. Alginate
2. Hydrocolloid
3. Hydrogel
4. Transparent film

2. When preparing to do a sterile dressing change, the nurse places sterile gauze pads on the sterile field but inadvertently touches the sterile field with an ungloved hand. Which of the following should the nurse do next?

1. Use only gauze pads from the sterile field away from the contaminated area.
2. Discard the gauze pads and sterile field and start over.
3. Continue with dressing change, as the gauze pads were not contaminated.
4. Place a new sterile field and using sterile gloves take gauze pads from the contaminated field and place on the new field.

3. What drip rate should the nurse set to deliver 1000 mL of intravenous D5W in 3 hours and 20 minutes if the drop factor is 15 drops per 1 mL? *Record your answer as a whole number.*

_____ drops/min

4. A client is taking the loop diuretic furosemide for edema associated with heart failure. Which electrolyte imbalance resulting from the medication is of most concern?

1. Hypokalemia
2. Hyperkalemia
3. Hypercalcemia
4. Hypocalcemia

5. Which of the following is the primary risk factor for cervical cancer?

1. Smoking
2. Chlamydia infection
3. Family history of cervical cancer
4. Human papillomavirus (HPV)

6. A 7-year-old child with special needs has difficulty learning activities that require more than one step. Which of the following approaches is likely to be the most effective?

1. Having the child master step one before progressing to step two
2. Coaching and assisting the child through each step sequentially
3. Providing posters with sequential pictures
4. Backward chaining

7. A client comes to a clinic with a severe cough and fever, but all of the exam rooms are full when the client arrives. Which of the following is the best action for the nurse to take?

1. Tell the client to reschedule an appointment for a less busy hour.
2. Ask the client to wait outside until an exam room becomes available.
3. Provide the client a facemask and seat her in the waiting area with other clients.
4. Provide the client a facemask and seat the client in a separate area as far as possible from other clients.

8. A mother brings her toddler to a well-baby clinic. The child is fair, and his skin is yellow-tinged, which is especially evident on his nose and the palms of his hands and feet. However, his sclerae are white. The nurse should anticipate that which of the following will be initially assessed?

1. Liver function tests
2. Diet
3. Blood count
4. Electrolytes

9. A client has had a pacemaker inserted recently but complains that he is experiencing heart palpitations, generalized weakness, and slight pain in the chest and jaw. On examination, the nurse notes that the client appears quite anxious, and the nurse observes pulsations in the neck and abdomen. Which of the following is the most likely cause of these findings?

1. Pacemaker wiring has become dislodged
2. Infection
3. Coronary artery occlusion
4. Pacemaker syndrome

10. A client has experienced a cardiac arrest at an office visit, and the nurse is going to administer defibrillation with an automated external defibrillator (AED). Which of the following should the nurse remove prior to administering a shock?

1. The client's watch
2. The client's bra with metal wires
3. The client's dentures
4. The client's nose ring

11. The mother of a 20-month-old child reports that another toddler in daycare developed a fever 7 days previously while in contact with the other children and subsequently was diagnosed with roseola. The mother is concerned that her child will develop roseola. What information should the nurse provide to the mother? *Select all that apply*.

1. Roseola is contagious with the onset of rash.
2. The incubation period for roseola is 9–10 days.
3. Roseola is contagious at the onset of fever.
4. The incubation period for roseola is 3–6 days.
5. Roseola is contagious 2 days prior to the onset of fever.

12. A client who has denied drug allergies has a telephone order for IM penicillin. Before the nurse administers the medication, the client states he thinks he may have developed a rash after "some drug." Which is the correct action?

1. Administer the drug and document a possible previous drug reaction.
2. Hold the drug and contact the prescribing physician.
3. Contact the pharmacist for guidance.
4. Contact the supervisor for guidance.

13. A 35-year-old woman is recovering from a thyroidectomy for Hashimoto's thyroiditis. The client complains that she is experiencing a tingling sensation about her mouth and fingers and muscle cramps in her legs. Which of the following complications is most likely the cause of these symptoms?

1. Hypocalcemia
2. Hypercalcemia
3. Hypermagnesemia
4. Hypomagnesemia

14. While observing the team leader irrigating a PICC line, a new nurse notes that the team leader has broken aseptic technique and contaminated the irrigating syringe. Which of the following actions is most appropriate?

1. Report the team leader to a supervisor.
2. Ask the team leader after the irrigation if sterile technique was required.
3. Say nothing because the new nurse is inexperienced.
4. Tell the team leader immediately that the irrigating syringe was contaminated.

15. A client with terminal cancer states she is not afraid of death but is afraid of the process of dying. Which of the following is the best response?

1. "What aspects of the dying process are you most concerned about?"
2. "Those are normal feelings."
3. "What can I do to help?"
4. "I'm so sorry."

16. A 70-year-old female states that she has difficulty falling asleep and sleeps poorly, often lying awake much of the night. The nurse should anticipate which of the following as the initial intervention?

1. Assessment of sleep patterns
2. Nocturnal polysomnogram
3. Prescription for hypnotic
4. Dietary modifications

17. The following ECG tracing is characteristic of which electrolyte imbalance?

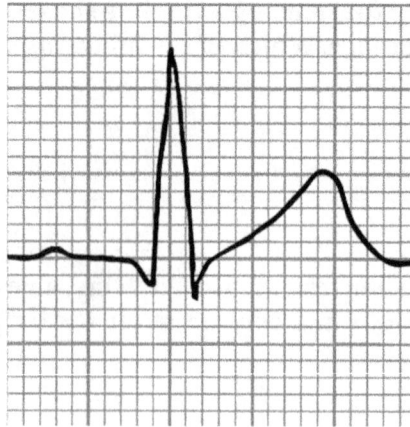

1. Hyperkalemia
2. Hypercalcemia
3. Hypomagnesemia
4. Hypermagnesemia

18. A client has had a stroke in the right hemisphere and has pronounced weakness on the left side and expressive aphasia. The nurse notes that the client has some dysphagia and is concerned that the client may aspirate. The nurse plans to ask the doctor about a referral to have the client's swallowing evaluated. The most appropriate referral is to which healthcare professional?

1. Speech and language therapist
2. Occupational therapist
3. Physical therapist
4. EENT specialist

19. The mother of an 11-year-old boy asks the nurse what type of anticipatory guidance she should provide for her son. Which of the following are age-appropriate topics the nurse should suggest for a child of this age? *Select all that apply.*

1. What to expect in terms of physical development and secondary sexual characteristics
2. Responsibilities of sexual behavior, including abstinence and birth control
3. Peer group pressures, including gangs, alcohol, and tobacco use
4. Future goals and plans
5. Dating and relationship issues

20. What is likely the cause of the following ECG tracing?

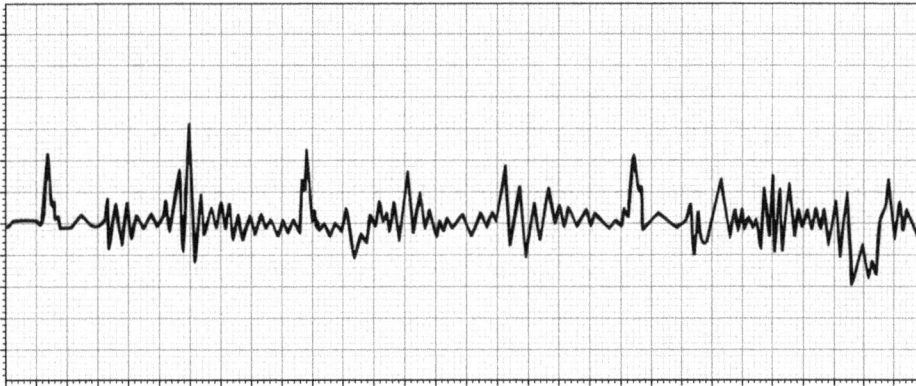

1. Electrical interference artifact
2. Dislodged electrode
3. Somatic tremor artifact
4. Broken recording

21. A client with dementia says to the nurse, "I'm going to the movies now. I always go to the movies on Thanksgiving evening. I hope it doesn't snow." Which is the most appropriate response?

1. "It's not Thanksgiving."
2. "What a lovely tradition! I love movies."
3. "Today is July 2. It's almost lunch time but after that you can watch a movie on TV."
4. "It's snowing, so this is not a good time to go to the movies."

22. A client with vaginal cancer is being treated with brachytherapy, and the nurse is explaining the procedure and precautions to the client. Which of the following information should the nurse include?

1. "Women who are pregnant and children under age 18 may not visit."
2. "Visitors should stay at least 2 feet away from the client."
3. "You can only leave your room for 5–10 minutes per day."
4. "Visitors can stay no more than 4 hours per day."

23. What does the ECG strip below indicate?

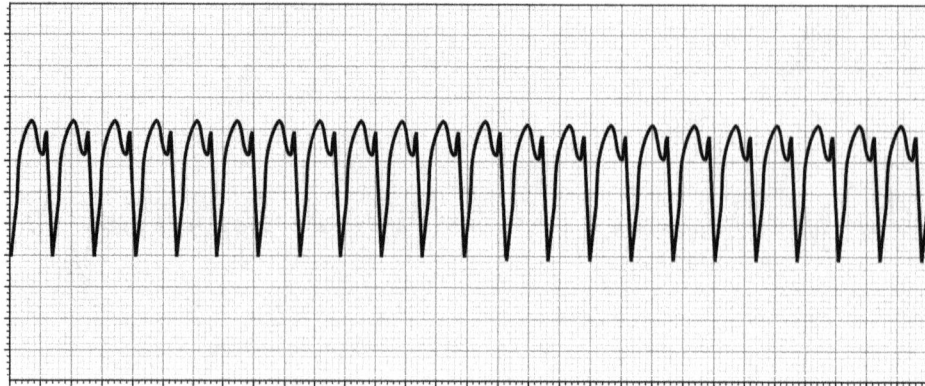

1. Ventricular paced rhythm
2. Supraventricular tachycardia
3. Atrial fibrillation
4. Ventricular tachycardia

24. A 26-year-old client is going to use continuous ambulatory peritoneal dialysis (CAPD) after discharge from the hospital. Which of the following should the nurse include in teaching about CAPD? *Select all that apply.*

1. "You will instill about 2 liters of fluid over 10–15 minutes."
2. "Clamp the tubing and maintain a dwell time of about 30 minutes."
3. "Unclamp the tubing and drain for about 20 minutes."
4. "Immerse the dialysate bag in warm water to increase temperature."
5. "You will instill about 2 liters of fluid over 3–5 hours."

25. The nurse is assisting a 19-year-old client who is not allowed to bear weight on his left foot when crutch walking, and the client states he wants to keep pace with his friends when they are walking. Which of the following crutch gaits requires the most energy but allows the fastest gait?

1. 4-point alternate
2. Swing-through
3. Swing-to
4. 2-point alternate

26. A 60-kilogram adult is to receive a medication that is administered at 0.5 mg per kg per 24 hours. If the medication is given in 2 equal doses (every 12 hours), how many milligrams should be in each dose? *Record your answer as a whole number.*

_____ mg

27. A 68-year-old client recently had a hip replacement for which she is receiving opioid analgesia. The patient refused dinner and exhibited sudden onset of weakness and confusion. During the assessment of the client, the nurse asks the client to show her teeth.

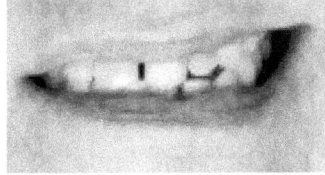

Based on the client's response (see photo), which of the following should the nurse expect as the *most* likely cause of the client's symptoms?

1. Over-medication
2. Hypoglycemia
3. Stroke
4. Delirium

28. The first-time mother of a 6-month-old infant is concerned that the child's physical development is delayed because the child cannot crawl. Which of the following is the most appropriate response?

1. "Most infants can crawl by 9 months."
2. "Most infants can crawl by 6 months."
3. "Don't worry, infants vary widely in abilities."
4. "Look at all your child can do!"

29. If a medication is available at 100 milligrams per 10 milliliters, how many milliliters does a dose of 120 milligrams require? *Record your answer as a whole number.*

_____ mL

30. A client has been on a weight-loss program. Her waist measures 28 inches, and her hips measure 40 inches. What is her waist-to-hip ratio? *Record your answer as a decimal.*

_____

31. The nurse is teaching a client with a sigmoid colostomy about colostomy care. Which of the following information should the nurse include? *Select all that apply.*

1. "You should expect to have a bowel movement every day."
2. "You may be able to regulate your bowel movements with diet or irrigations."
3. "Your stool may be soft to solid."
4. "There are different types of colostomy appliances available."
5. "Your stool will probably be semi-liquid."

32. A client receiving total parenteral nutrition (TPN) must receive 2 grams of protein per kilogram of body weight per day. The patient weighs 136.4 pounds. How many total grams of protein should the client receive each day? *Record your answer as a whole number.*

_____ grams

33. What does the small positive deflection (indicated by the arrow) represent?

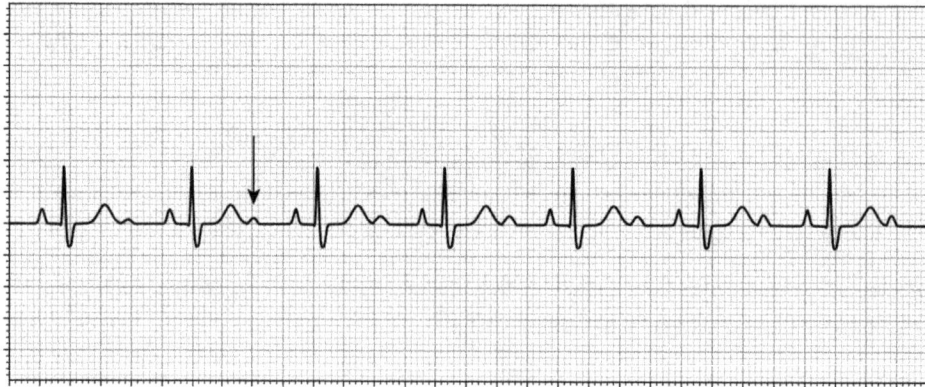

1. Notched T wave
2. Artifact
3. Premature P wave
4. U wave

34. The nurse is using motivational interviewing with a client who is addicted to heroin to change behaviors. Which of the following are important elements of motivational interviewing? *Select all that apply.*

1. Express empathy instead of criticism.
2. Focus on the client's weaknesses.
3. Avoid confrontation.
4. Listen instead of giving advice.
5. Actively oppose client resistance.

35. A client is receiving a liter of normal saline intravenously but must receive 150 mL of antibiotic solution by piggyback. Which of the following is the most correct procedure?

1. Clamp the primary tubing and adjust the flow rate of the piggyback unit.
2. Hang the piggyback unit 6 inches lower than the primary unit and adjust flow rate of the piggyback unit only.
3. Hang the piggyback unit 6 inches higher than the primary unit and adjust flow rate of the piggyback unit only.
4. Hang the piggyback unit at the same level as the primary unit, clamp the primary tubing, and adjust flow rate of the piggyback unit.

36. When conducting a physical examination of a 62-year-old female, the nurse notes nodules on the dorsolateral aspects of the distal interphalangeal joints (Heberden's nodes) of the right hand. Which of the following diseases does this finding suggest?

1. Acute tenosynovitis
2. Gout
3. Rheumatoid arthritis
4. Osteoarthritis

37. A client experiences a severe generalized tonic-clonic seizure while in bed in supine position with one side rail down. Which of the following actions by the nurse are correct? *Select all that apply.*

1. Insert a padded tongue blade between the client's teeth.
2. Turn the client to the side-lying position.
3. Elevate and pad the side rails.
4. Leave the side rail down and stand on the open side to restrain the client if needed.
5. Restrain the patient physically throughout the seizure.

38. Which vitamin or mineral may alter the effect of levodopa in clients treated for Parkinson's disease?

1. Calcium
2. Vitamin D
3. Ascorbic acid (vitamin C)
4. Pyridoxine (vitamin B6)

39. A client with osteomyelitis of the right tibia that has cultured positive for *Staphylococcus aureus* is to be discharged home with dressing changes done daily by nurses from a home health agency. When teaching family members about infection control, which of the following is the most important point to stress?

1. Limiting contact with others
2. Sterilizing environmental surfaces
3. Wearing gowns and gloves for all contact with the client
4. Handwashing

40. What is the approximate duration of the QRS complex on the ECG tracing below?

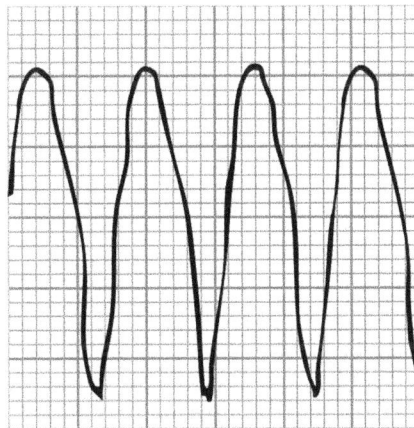

1. 0.28 s
2. 0.32 s
3. 0.36 s
4. 0.40 s

41. The nurse is teaching a newly diagnosed client with diabetes mellitus type 1 about self-care. Which of the following information should the nurse include? *Select all that apply*.

1. Glucose testing
2. Skin care
3. Dietary compliance
4. Bowel care
5. Insulin administration

42. Which of the following blood products is indicated for a client with disseminated intravascular coagulation (DIC) to control bleeding where replacement of coagulation factors is necessary?

1. Whole blood
2. Irradiated red blood cells
3. Fresh frozen plasma
4. Platelets (multiple donors)

43. The nurse is a member of a team in which two members have an escalating personal conflict that is affecting team morale and functioning. Which of the following initial responses is most appropriate?

1. Tell the two members they are acting childishly.
2. Report the two members to the unit supervisor.
3. Express concern and offer to mediate.
4. Ignore the situation as much as possible.

44. A client has requested pain medication, but after the nurse obtains the prescribed dose of codeine from the dispensing cart, the client refuses to take the medication, stating he might want it later. What should the nurse do with the medication?

1. Return it to the dispensing cart.
2. Leave it at the client's bedside.
3. Dispose of the medication according to facility protocol with two appropriate witnesses.
4. Place the medication in a tray for later use.

45. The nurse observed another nurse remove a hydrocodone tablet from a client's medicine drawer and then swallow the tablet when it appeared no one was looking. Which of the following is the most appropriate response?

1. Immediately report the incident to a direct supervisor.
2. Immediately confront the nurse.
3. Report the incident to the police.
4. Report the incident to the client's physician.

46. An adolescent was struck by a car and brought to the emergency room unconscious. Because he was not carrying an ID, the nurse has been unable to locate a parent or family member to provide consent. The client has a ruptured spleen, and the physician states the client needs immediate life-saving surgery. The nurse should:

1. Contact administration for a consent waiver.
2. Hold the client's transfer until a family member is found.
3. Sign the consent form since no one else is available to do so.
4. Transfer the client to surgery without a consent form signed.

47. A client is scheduled to undergo a cholecystectomy. Which of the following is a required element of informed consent?

1. Duration of operation
2. Names of surgical staff
3. Risks and benefits
4. Insurance coverage

48. A woman comes to the emergency department after being badly beaten. She is shaking and appears very frightened. Which of the following is the first question the nurse should ask?

1. "Who did this to you?"
2. "Is the person who did this to you present here in the hospital?"
3. "Have you called the police?"
4. "Do you want information about women's shelters?"

49. A client has been recovering well from a knee replacement but has a sudden onset of restlessness and anxiety. The client complains of chest pain, shortness of breath, and a cough with frothy, blood-tinged sputum. The client has a pulse of 110 bpm and a temperature of 101.2 °F (38.4 °C). The nurse notes rales in the right lung and tachypnea. Based on these findings, which of the following complications is most likely?

1. Pulmonary embolism
2. Atelectasis
3. Pneumonia
4. Pneumothorax

50. Which of the following laboratory findings are consistent with hypernatremia?

1. Increased serum sodium and decreased urine sodium
2. Increased serum sodium and decreased urine osmolality
3. Increased serum sodium and increased urine sodium
4. Increased serum sodium and decreased urine specific gravity

51. A client with diabetes has been advised by the physician to do strength training twice a week and to engage in aerobic activities. The client has indicated an interest in walking, which is a moderate aerobic exercise. How many minutes per week should the client be advised to walk to meet current exercise guidelines? *Record your answer as a whole number.*

_____ minutes

52. The nurse is working in the emergency department when a multi-car accident occurs on a nearby interstate highway, resulting in many casualties. The following injured people are the first to arrive:

> I. 64-year-old female, alert and responsive, with a large laceration on the head
> II. 16-year-old male with a chest injury who is in respiratory distress and severe pain
> III. 28-year-old male with multiple contusions and a fractured right arm
> IV. Middle-aged male with unknown injuries who is very agitated, hallucinating, confused, and reeking of alcohol

If carrying out triage and considering the severity of injury, in which order (indicating with the corresponding Roman numeral) should the clients be treated?

1. _____
2. _____
3. _____
4. _____

53. A client is recovering from abdominal surgery after a gunshot wound. When the nurse sees increased sanguineous drainage and changes the dressing, the nurse notes that the midline abdominal incision is dehiscing and a loop of the intestine has eviscerated through the lower third of the wound. While the client is awaiting transfer to surgery for repair, which of the following interventions should the nurse carry out? *Select all that apply.*

1. Wearing sterile gloves, attempt to reinsert the viscera through the open wound.
2. Cover the viscera with a dry sterile dressing.
3. Cover the viscera with a normal saline–soaked sterile dressing.
4. Place the client in low Fowler's position with knees slightly flexed.
5. Place the client in Trendelenburg position.

54. The nurse notes that a portable electrocardiogram machine that is in frequent use has a frayed electrical cord. Which of the following is the most appropriate initial response?

1. Place tape around the frayed section of cord.
2. Tape a "beware frayed cord" notice to the machine.
3. Immediately remove the machine from service.
4. Notify the unit supervisor that the machine needs repair.

55. A nurse assesses a patient's IV site and notes slight swelling around the insertion site. The skin is cool to touch and the patient verbalizes discomfort. The nurse identifies this as most likely being:

1. Phlebitis
2. Infiltration
3. Extravasation
4. Infection

56. A client with asthma is to be discharged and must take nebulizer treatments at home. Which of the following is the best method to ensure that the client understands how to use and clean the equipment after the nurse completes a demonstration?

1. Provide the client with written instructions.
2. Provide the client with a telephone number to call if questions arise.
3. Ask the client if he has any questions.
4. Ask the client to do a return demonstration.

57. A pregnant woman at 21 weeks gestation has severe preeclampsia with a BP of 170/120 and proteinuria of 6 g in 24 hours. What treatment should the nurse anticipate is initially indicated?

1. Bedrest only
2. Phenytoin
3. Magnesium sulfate
4. Antihypertensive, such as hydralazine

58. Fetal heart tones are usually first heard with a fetoscope at what week of gestation? *Record your answer as a whole number.*

_____

59. A client complains of blurred vision, fatigue, loss of appetite, weight loss, increased thirst, and frequent urination. Which of the following laboratory assessment(s) would be most indicated?

1. Blood glucose and HbA1c
2. Serum and urine osmolality
3. Complete blood count
4. Urinalysis

60. A neonate has hyperbilirubinemia and jaundice, and the physician has prescribed phototherapy, which the nurse is about to administer.

I. Place a protective mask over the child's eyes.
II. Adjust the light source to 15–20 cm above the child.
III. Turn on lights.
IV. Remove all clothes except diaper.

Place the actions listed above (Roman numerals) in order, beginning with the first action.

1. _____
2. _____
3. _____
4. _____

61. According to USDA dietary guidelines depicted in the diagram, which of the following meals most closely corresponds to dietary recommendations?

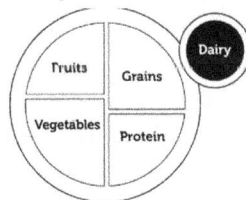

1. 1 apple, 1 cup of carrots, 1 cup of long-grain white rice, 4 ounces of poached salmon, and 1 half-cup of sweetened yogurt
2. 1 cup of canned fruit cocktail, 1 cup of corn, 1 cup of long-grain white rice, 4 ounces of fried breaded fish sticks, and 8 ounces of wine
3. 1 cup of steamed kale, 1 medium baked potato with butter and sour cream, 6 ounces of rib-eye steak, and 1 cup of coffee
4. Half of a banana, 1 cup of broccoli, 1 half-cup of quinoa, 3 ounces of roasted turkey, and 8 ounces of 1% milk

62. When teaching a client with a seizure disorder about the long-term use of phenytoin, the nurse should stress the necessity for which of the following? *Select all that apply.*

1. Dental care
2. Hearing examinations
3. Vitamin D therapy and evaluation for osteoporosis
4. Drug compliance
5. Regular exercise

63. A client is treated in the emergency department for second-degree burns after falling asleep while sunbathing. The client states she sunbathes 8–10 hours every week to maintain a tan. Which of the following advice is most important to share with the client? *Select all that apply.*

1. Excessive exposure to the sun increases the risk of skin cancer.
2. The client should limit tanning to 2–3 hours at a time.
3. Self-tanners are available that do not require sun exposure.
4. There is no value in exposing the skin to the sun.
5. Sunscreen should be applied for prolonged exposure to the sun.

64. A 68-year-old client states he decided not to take the herpes zoster (shingles) immunization because his friend had the immunization and still developed shingles. Which of the following information should the nurse include when discussing this issue with the client? *Select all that apply.*

1. Shingles rarely occurs after immunization.
2. The immunization decreases the severity of infection.
3. The immunization decreases the likelihood of postherpetic syndrome.
4. The immunization cuts the chance of developing shingles in half.
5. The client should never take advice from friends.

65. A client who received an IV antibiotic mistakenly believed she was receiving opioid analgesia and reported a few minutes later that the medication had relieved her pain. Which of the following is the most likely reason for the client's response?

1. The client was lying about having pain.
2. The antibiotic actually relieved the pain.
3. The client experienced a placebo effect.
4. The client's pain subsided coincidentally.

66. A female client complains of a sudden onset of chest and abdominal "tightness" and pressure with pain in the neck and jaw. The client feels fatigued and nauseated. She appears pale and dyspneic, and her skin is cold and clammy. Which of the following diagnostic tests should the nurse anticipate will be completed initially?

1. Electrocardiogram
2. Bronchoscopy
3. Echocardiogram
4. Complete blood count

67. The nurse is serving on the performance improvement committee, which has agreed to some changes in procedures on the basis of evidence-based research. If the committee wants to convince staff members to comply with the changes, which of the following actions should the committee carry out first?

1. Identify and gain support of key staff.
2. Explain the consequences of failure to comply.
3. Determine a reward system for compliance.
4. Clearly outline expectations in written format.

68. A client with a large pressure injury is suffering from malnutrition and has had little protein in her diet. What effect does inadequate protein intake have on wound healing?

1. It has little or no effect.
2. It inhibits phagocytosis of white blood cells.
3. It slows the healing process because of the lack of amino acids.
4. It causes vasoconstriction that impairs circulation.

69. A client in the cardiac care unit has been very upset since two other clients in the unit died and tells the nurse, "Everyone dies here. I don't know why you are bothering treating me." Which of the following is the most therapeutic response?

1. "You are worried that you're going to die."
2. "You are recovering well, so you don't need to worry."
3. "The other clients were much sicker than you are."
4. "You should discuss your concerns with your doctor."

70. The rhythm on the following ECG tracing would be interpreted as:

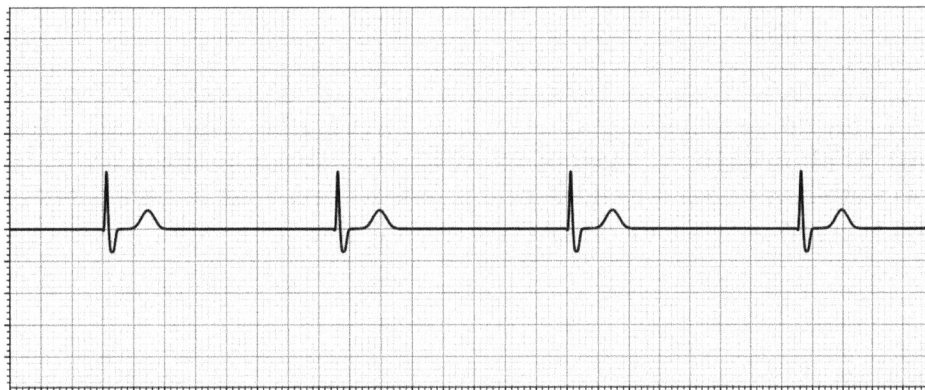

1. Sinus bradycardia
2. First-degree heart block
3. Junctional escape rhythm
4. Wandering atrial pacemaker

71. A nurse has delegated a task to a fellow nurse. After delegating, the delegating nurse's responsibility is to

1. Leave the task and outcomes to the fellow nurse to monitor.
2. Ask the fellow nurse if the task was completed.
3. Assume the task was completed and document accordingly.
4. Follow up to ensure the task was completed and outcomes were appropriate.

72. Describe the duration, amplitude, and appearance of the P waves in the following ECG tracing:

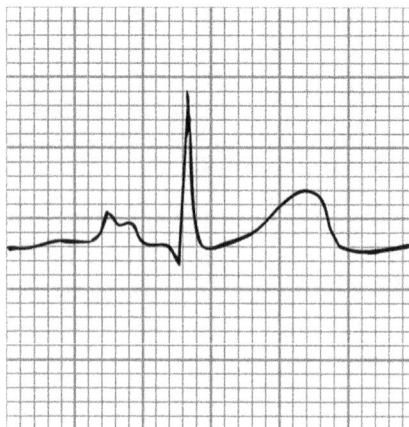

1. 0.28 s, 3 mm, rounded
2. 0.09 s, 2 mm, peaked
3. 0.12 s, 1 mm, notched
4. 0.12 s, 2 mm, notched

73. A client has had three recent bouts of cystitis and now has urinary frequency and burning, chills, a fever of 102 °F (38.9 °C), abdominal pain, and bilateral flank pain. Which of the following diagnostic tests should the nurse expect the physician to order initially?

1. Complete blood count
2. Urinalysis and urine culture and sensitivities
3. Kidney function tests
4. Cystoscopy

74. A client tells the nurse that she has always hated her mother, who left the client behind with her abusive father when the parents divorced. The mother has been trying to reestablish a relationship with the client, who is now 23 years old, but the client remains uncertain and angry. Which spiritual need is the client grappling with?

1. Love
2. Faith
3. Hope
4. Forgiveness

75. A client is admitted to a drug rehabilitation program. He appears thin with scattered lesions where he has been picking at his skin and shows evidence of severe tooth decay. He is very talkative and has a rapid, irregular heartbeat. Based on these signs and symptoms, which of the following is most likely his drug of choice?

1. Cocaine
2. Methamphetamine
3. Marijuana
4. LSD

76. A client has stage 4 pancreatic cancer and is taking high doses of morphine to control severe pain. Which statement by the client's spouse and caregiver suggests a need for education?

1. "The morphine doesn't seem to be working as well now."
2. "I think death will be a relief for both of us."
3. "This experience has shaken my belief in God."
4. "I know all this morphine is making her a drug addict."

77. What rhythm is evident on this ECG strip?

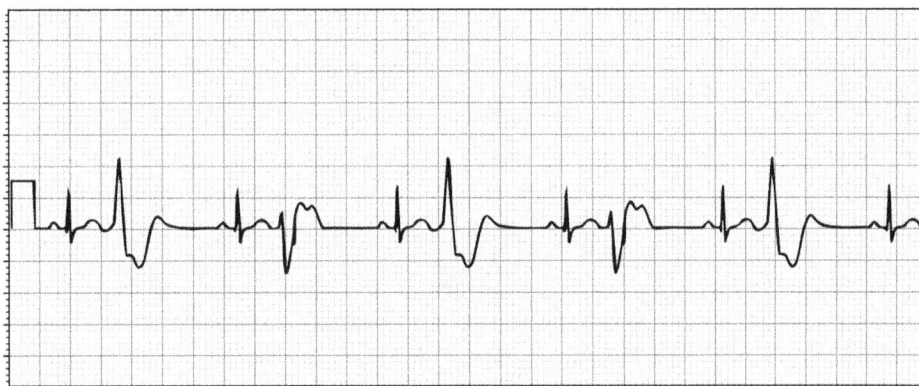

1. AV block (Mobitz I)
2. Atrial bigeminy
3. Ventricular escape beats
4. PVC and ventricular bigeminy

78. A home care client has been having an Unna boot replaced every 7 days, but at a home visit, the nurse finds the patient cannot ambulate because of an injury to the opposite leg. Which of the following actions is most correct at this time?

1. The Unna boot should be discontinued and the leg left open.
2. The Unna boot should be changed as scheduled.
3. The Unna boot should be discontinued and replaced with a short stretch wrap (such as Comprilan).
4. The Unna boot should be discontinued and another form of compression used.

79. A client on cardiac monitoring has dislodged his leads 6 times in a 4-hour period, setting off alarms. Each time, he makes a different excuse, but the nurse suspects the dislodgements are purposeful because the client attempts to delay the nurse's leaving after each episode. Which of the following is the most appropriate response?

1. "I can see that you are doing this on purpose."
2. "These constant alarms are disturbing to other patients."
3. "Why are you disconnecting your leads?"
4. "Let's talk about the reason for monitoring and what we can learn from it."

80. Which of the following is the most effective scale for assessing pain in a 6-year-old child?

1. Wong-Baker FACES pain scale
2. 0-10 numeric pain intensity scale
3. PAINAD scale
4. CRIES scale

81. A patient had a bowel resection and has been reluctant to take deep breaths and cough because of discomfort. Which of the following interventions is most indicated initially to prevent atelectasis?

1. Regular use of incentive spirometer
2. Nebulizer treatments with albuterol
3. IPPB treatments
4. Prophylactic antibiotics

82. The nurse is discussing the use of a condom with a sexually active 17-year-old male client being treated for gonorrhea. Which of the following information should the nurse include? *Select all that apply.*

1. Use a condom every time for every sexual encounter.
2. Use natural membrane condoms, which provide better protection than latex.
3. Use only water-based lubricants.
4. Hold the condom in place when withdrawing the penis after ejaculation.
5. Apply the condom so it fits snugly against the glans of the penis.

83. A client is admitted to the hospital from a board-and-care facility with a coccygeal pressure injury that is 5 by 8 cm in size, involves partial thickness loss of dermis, and has a red/pink wound surface without slough. Based on these observations, what stage is the pressure injury?

1. Stage I
2. Stage II
3. Stage III
4. Stage IV

84. A client is receiving radiotherapy to the abdominal area and has developed chronic diarrhea. Which of the following should the nurse include when teaching the client ways to manage the diarrhea? *Select all that apply.*

1. "It's important to drink 8–12 glasses of clear fluids each day."
2. "It's better to eat 5 or 6 small meals than 3 large meals."
3. "Try to increase the fiber in your diet."
4. "You can try the BRAT diet (banana, rice, applesauce, and toast)."
5. "Drinking milk and eating ice cream may soothe your stomach."

85. A client tells the nurse that his physician has advised him to take over-the-counter (OTC) anti-inflammatory drugs to control the discomfort of osteoarthritis. The client asks the nurse what drugs to consider. Which of the following medications should the nurse advise the client are OTC anti-inflammatory drugs? *Select all that apply.*

1. NSAIDs
2. Corticosteroids
3. Acetaminophen
4. Salicylates

86. A full-term pregnant woman experienced premature rupture of the membranes 24 hours earlier but has not gone into labor. Which of the following should the nurse anticipate?

1. Labor will be induced.
2. The client is at increased risk of hemorrhage.
3. The client will undergo a Caesarean.
4. Labor will be induced if the patient does not go into labor within 48 hours.

87. The nurse is completing a physical examination of a client and evaluating the client for peripheral arterial and venous insufficiency. Which of the following findings are consistent with peripheral arterial insufficiency? *Select all that apply*.

1. Brownish discoloration appears about the ankles and anterior tibial area.
2. The foot exhibits rubor on dependency and pallor on elevation.
3. Ulcers are evident on the end of the great toe and heel.
4. Peripheral edema is marked.
5. Ulcers are superficial and irregular, often on medial or lateral malleolus.

88. When taking an adult client's blood pressure, the lower border of the cuff should be how far above the antecubital crease?

1. 1 cm
2. 5 cm
3. 2.5 cm
4. 7.5 cm

89. A female client's CBC showed the following results:

Test	Result	
WBC	4.1	$10^3/\mu L$
RBC	4.38	$10^6/\mu L$
Hemoglobin	13.8	g/dL
Hematocrit	42	%
Platelet count	116	$10^3/\mu L$

Which of the tests are outside of the normal range?

1. Hemoglobin and hematocrit
2. All tests
3. Platelet count and WBC
4. Platelet count and RBC

90. The ECG changes that are seen with both myocardial injury and myocardial infarction include:

1. ST-segment elevation and T-wave inversion
2. ST-segment depression and T-wave inversion
3. Prolonged QT segment with T-wave inversion
4. T-wave inversion and absent P wave

91. What is notable about the ECG tracing below?

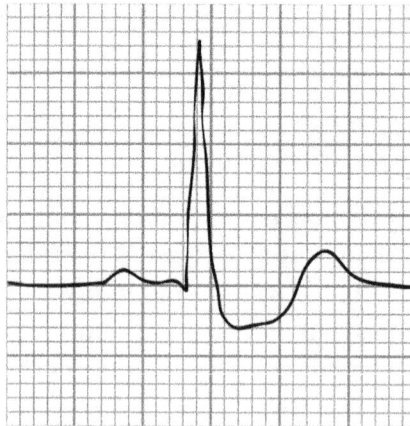

1. Prolonged P wave
2. Narrow QRS complex
3. ST segment elevation
4. ST segment depression

92. A 5-year-old child is undergoing chemotherapy for acute lymphocytic leukemia (ALL). The child comes into a clinic for weekly blood tests to monitor status. Which of the following abnormalities of the blood are of most concern during treatment for leukemia?

1. Thrombocytopenia and neutropenia
2. Thrombocytosis and neutropenia
3. Thrombocytosis and neutrocytosis
4. Thrombocytopenia and neutrocytosis

93. The nurse is interviewing a 56-year-old male with obstructive sleep apnea (OSA) for which he has been prescribed a CPAP machine for use during sleep. The client yawns frequently during the interview. Which of the following statements by the client indicates a need for further education about OSA and CPAP?

1. "I use only distilled water for humidification."
2. "I try to use the CPAP most nights."
3. "I wash the mask and tubing with soap and water and rinse with water and vinegar."
4. "I think the nasal mask is better than the orofacial mask."

94. The nurse is floated to the oncology unit but has not had previous experience administering IV chemotherapy, which the nurse must administer to two clients. Which of the following is the most appropriate response?

1. Research the drugs and correct administration prior to giving them.
2. Ask one of the other nurses to assist with administration.
3. Discuss the lack of experience with the unit supervisor.
4. Refuse to administer the chemotherapy.

95. The nurse must move a patient who is lying supine onto the side of the bed in preparation for transfer to a wheelchair. The steps to this procedure include the following:

I. Roll the client onto their side, facing the nurse.

II. Place one hand under the shoulders and the other over the hips.

III. Raise the head of the bed to 30°.

IV. Pivot the client into a sitting position.

Place the steps (in Roman numerals) into the correct order:

1. ____
2. ____
3. ____
4. ____

96. A client receiving digoxin exhibits tachycardia and complains of headache, fatigue, nausea, diarrhea, and halo vision. Which of the following is probably the cause?

1. Digoxin dosage too low
2. An allergic response to digoxin
3. Digoxin toxicity
4. Disorder unrelated to digoxin

97. How long should a woman remain in the supine position after administration of a vaginal suppository?

1. 1–2 minutes
2. 3–5 minutes
3. 5–10 minutes
4. 15 minutes

98. The nurse must administer eye drops to a 6-month-old infant, but the child clinches the eyes tightly to avoid the drops. Which of the following actions is the most appropriate?

1. Attempt to instill the drops at a later time.
2. Force the infant's eyes open using the thumb and index finger.
3. Gently restrain the head and apply the drops at the inner canthus.
4. Pull down the lower lid with the thumb and instill the drops into the conjunctival sac.

99. A 36-year-old woman who smokes 2 packs of cigarettes daily seeks advice about contraception. Which of the following contraceptive methods should she avoid? *Select all that apply.*

1. Vaginal ring
2. Combined hormone pills
3. Intrauterine device
4. Progestin-only pill
5. All contraceptives except condoms and diaphragms

100. The slurred upstroke of the QRS complex in this ECG waveform is referred to as a(n):

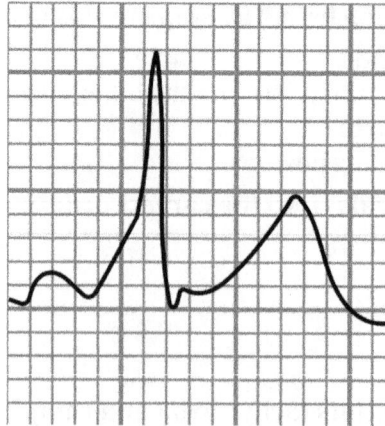

1. De Winter's sign
2. Spodick's sign
3. Epsilon wave
4. Delta wave

Answer Key and Explanations for Test #1

Case Study 1

1. 2, 3, 5, and 6: Whenever a client admits to taking too much of any medication, it is important to know how much was taken and when it was taken. This allows the medical team to estimate how long the client needs to be monitored for adverse symptoms. The maximum acetaminophen dose for the average adult is 4,000 mg, and the client has surpassed this. This is also evident with the client's elevated serum acetaminophen level. The client's history of depression and previous suicide attempts put her at a greater risk of reattempting suicide, meaning the client should be closely monitored and anything potentially harmful should be removed from her room. Her blood ethanol being elevated is also concerning because it can exacerbate the acetaminophen's hepatotoxic properties. The client's ALT/AST levels are currently normal, but she should continue to be monitored because her liver function may worsen as the acetaminophen is metabolized. The client's heart rate and respiratory rate are slightly elevated, but this is likely caused by anxiety. The nurse should monitor for the worsening of these symptoms.

2. 4: Because acetaminophen is metabolized in the liver, an overdose can add increased strain, which can lead to acute-onset liver failure. Cirrhosis is the scarring of the liver that is a result of chronic liver injury, often secondary to alcohol abuse. Over time, cirrhosis can lead to chronic liver failure rather than the acute-onset liver failure experienced secondary to acetaminophen toxicity. Kidney failure and GI bleeds are less likely to happen with acetaminophen overdose, but they may happen with nonsteroidal anti-inflammatory drug (such as ibuprofen or aspirin) overdoses. However, a GI bleed could potentially occur secondary to liver failure due to changes in platelet production and secondary conditions such as portal hypertension.

3.

- Place on a mental health hold.
- Administer IV ondansetron.
- Obtain urinary toxicology.
- Administer IV acetylcysteine.
- Obtain a bedside urine pregnancy test.

Placing the client on a mental health hold and administering IV acetylcysteine are both of the highest priority because they are time sensitive and are related to the client's safety and health outcomes. Acetylcysteine acts to counter the hepatotoxic effects of the acetaminophen overdose. When an overdose is identified (usually through elevated serum acetaminophen levels), acetylcysteine should be administered as soon as possible to prevent liver damage. The mental health hold orders will involve collaboration with the mental health team and will provide resources to ensure the client's safety. Administering IV ondansetron may also be done to decrease the client's discomfort with nausea, but it is unlikely to change the overall outcomes. Obtaining urine toxicology should also be done in case there are additional drugs in the client's system causing her symptoms, but this is not as emergent or time sensitive. A urine pregnancy test may also be necessary to inform the client's care, but it is not as emergent or time sensitive as the aforementioned priorities.

33

4.

Potential Nursing Interventions	Indicated	Not Indicated
Request an order for repeat labs in 4 hours.	●	○
Place the client on seizure precautions.	○	●
Contact the local poison control center.	●	○
Notify the mental health team and charge nurse that the client is suicidal.	●	○
Remove cardiac monitoring from the room.	○	●
Ask the client's visitor to leave.	○	●

Repeat liver function and acetaminophen labs should be collected within 4–6 hours of acetaminophen overdose to monitor for signs of liver damage and for signs that the acetaminophen is being metabolized (or not). A resource such as the local poison control center or a toxicologist should be contacted whenever a client overdoses on medication to ensure that the health team is monitoring the client for expected symptoms and on how best to treat the overdose. It is important to supply information such as the time of ingestion, amount ingested, and the age of the client. The mental health team and unit leadership should be notified as soon as possible that the client is suicidal so that safety measures can be put in place and so the mental health team can be present for further evaluation when the client is medically cleared. These safety measures may vary between facilities, but they often include removing the client's belongings, providing alternative clothing, removing potentially dangerous objects from the room, and providing a sitter who can ensure that the client does not try to leave or harm him-/herself. Seizure precautions are not generally indicated for acetaminophen overdoses but may be indicated for other overdoses such as antihistamines or antidepressants. Although the cords for cardiac monitoring may be considered a potential suicide hazard, their removal should be weighed based on the need to monitor the client and the likelihood that she will impulsively harm herself with them. In this case, the client has supportive family present, has contracted to safety, and needs to have cardiac monitoring due to a drug overdose. In some cases, it may be necessary to remove a mental health client's visitor because the visitor may exacerbate the client's mental health symptoms. However, in this case, the visitor is presenting as a support system for the client and could help improve the client's willingness to participate in care and help her feel safer and more comfortable in the stressful hospital environment.

5.

Assessment Findings	Improved	Unchanged	Worsened
GI symptoms	●	○	○
Liver function	○	○	●
Blood pressure, 115/85	○	●	○
Serum acetaminophen	●	○	○

The client is no longer feeling nauseous and has an improved appetite, which are signs that her GI symptoms have improved. Additionally, her serum acetaminophen levels have decreased, which is an improvement and a sign that it is being metabolized. These levels should continue to be

34

monitored throughout her care. Her liver function, as shown with increased AST and ALT, has worsened. This lab result should be given to the client's physician immediately for potential further treatment. The client's blood pressure is still within the normal range and thus is considered unchanged.

6. 2, 3, and 5: It is true that the client's liver function will need to be monitored for the duration of her hospitalization because the signs of damage from acetaminophen overdose may not be present until hours or even days later. Additionally, once she is deemed to no longer need medical monitoring or treatment, the client will likely be evaluated by the mental health team and could be sent to a mental health facility for further acute treatment. The exact process may vary somewhat depending on the state, the facility, and what resources are available. Although the client on a mental health hold may not leave the hospital until a physician or mental health professional deems it safe for her to do so, the client still has human rights. It is important that these rights are expressed to the client. The person who reads these rights to the client may be the nurse, a physician, or a mental health professional depending on the facility and on the state of residence. It is also important to show the client that she is not considered "crazy" for her mental health emergency. Padded rooms, isolation, and restraints should be used rarely and only if the client is in imminent danger of harming herself or others.

Case Study 2

1. 2 and 7: The client's reddish-purple rash and bruising are new findings that warrant further investigation. The client's complaint of metallic taste and numbness/tingling to his feet and hands and observed pallor remain stable and his fatigue is not limiting ADLs at this time. These side effects should continue to be monitored but are not a priority concern. The client's blood pressure is low, but it is not at a concerning level.

2. 1: The rash (petechiae) and bruising (ecchymosis) are symptoms associated with thrombocytopenia. Neutropenia and anemia likely explain the pallor and fatigue, which are not new findings. The patient is not described as being cachectic (experiencing unintended weight loss).

3. 4: A platelet count of 19,000/μL is significantly low and is the likely cause of the client's petechiae (rash) and ecchymosis (bruising). Although the other findings are also low, none directly correlate with the client's new symptoms.

4.

Potential Medical Interventions	Indicated	Not Indicated
Arrange for a repeat CBC and nurse visit in 24 hours.	●	○
Administer IV antiemetics.	○	●
Administer IV platelets.	●	○
Administer subcutaneous heparin.	○	●
Hold cycle five of chemotherapy.	●	○

The oncologist would advise the nurse to administer IV platelets to boost the client's current platelet count and to hold this cycle of treatment until the platelet count shows improvement. The oncologist would want to closely monitor the client with a repeat CBC and nurse evaluation within the next day or two. Antiemetics are not needed because the client does not complain of nausea or vomiting. Heparin would be contraindicated at this time due to the client's risk for bleeding.

5.

- Avoid crowded places.
- Use a soft-bristled toothbrush.
- Use an electric razor.
- Take breaks between ADLs.
- Go to the ED if experiencing a nosebleed that will not stop.
- Take ibuprofen or naproxen for a headache.

A soft-bristled toothbrush is recommended to prevent bleeding gums, and an electric razor helps prevent cuts when shaving. The client would be encouraged to go to the ED for emergent evaluation and treatment for a nosebleed that does not stop after a few minutes, as this would indicate that his platelet count is critically low. Avoiding crowded places and taking breaks during ADLs are not necessary actions. Ibuprofen and naproxen are contraindicated because they prevent platelet aggregation.

6.

Assessment Findings	Improved	Unchanged	Worsened
Spontaneously bleeding gums	○	○	●
Light rash on the bilateral feet	●	○	○
Eraser tip-sized black spot on the tongue	○	●	○
Sudden sharp headache	○	○	●
Platelet count 20,000/µL	○	●	○

The client's condition has improved if the rash has diminished, indicating no further capillary hemorrhage in the lower extremities. A small black spot on the tongue is a bruise similar to that previously noted on the client's arm, which indicates no change in the client's condition. The platelet count of 20,000/µL is essentially the same as the previous lab value. Bleeding gums that are not caused by injury indicate a low platelet count and an inability to clot. A sudden sharp headache is a medical emergency that indicates a possible brain hemorrhage.

Case Study 3

1. 1, 2, 5, 6, and 7: The nurse should follow up on symptoms of a potential cardiac problem (epigastric pain and diaphoresis) and signs of altered perfusion (elevated heart rate, decreased blood pressure, and tachypnea) due to the risk of serious injury or even death to the client. Although the client is hypoxic and tachypneic, his lung sounds are normal and do not require follow-up at this time. Although his bowel sounds should be monitored going forward, they would not be a priority for follow-up with the existence of more urgent symptoms.

2.

Client Findings	MI	SIRS	Cardiogenic Shock
Epigastric pain	■	□	□
Diaphoresis	■	□	□
Restlessness	■	■	■
Nausea	■	□	□
Heart rate, 120	□	■	■

The client is presenting with several symptoms of an MI, including radiating chest pain (sometimes described by clients as epigastric pain), diaphoresis, restlessness, and nausea. Although not always present, clients will also commonly experience tachycardia when having an MI due to anxiety, pain, or the strain placed on the heart. In order to be diagnosed with SIRS, a client must have at least two of the following four symptoms: tachycardia, tachypnea, alteration in normal temperature (either fever or hypothermia), and alteration in white blood cell count (either >12,000/mm^3 or <4,000/mm^3). Restlessness can also be present due to the systemic effects of SIRS. Cardiogenic shock is a result of such severe damage to the heart that it can no longer adequately supply the body with blood and oxygen, resulting in symptoms such as tachycardia, hypotension, tachypnea, and restlessness. Although cardiogenic shock can be due to a heart attack, it can also be caused by chronic conditions such as congestive heart failure, and it is not always associated with acute cardiac symptoms such as chest pain.

3. 2: The client is demonstrating the signs of cardiogenic shock, which can rapidly progress to cardiac arrest due to lack of perfusion to the heart. Although a client may develop heart failure if the heart suffers permanent damage from an MI, this would be a long-term problem and would not be the most immediate risk to the client. A pneumothorax develops when air enters the pleural space and places pressure on the lung, causing it to collapse. This is most often caused by trauma or surgery that allows air to enter the pleural space and is not the most immediate risk to the client.

4.

Potential Nursing Interventions	Indicated	Not Indicated
Apply automatic external defibrillator pads, one to the upper right side of the chest and one to the lower left lateral side of the chest.	●	○
Administer a sublingual nitroglycerin 0.3 mg tablet per the facility's cardiac arrest protocol.	○	●
Apply a nonrebreather oxygen mask at 10 L/min.	○	●
Activate a code blue.	●	○
Begin chest compressions at 120 beats per minute.	●	○
Place the client in the semi-Fowler's position.	○	●

The client is experiencing cardiac arrest; it is essential that the nurse begin compressions and activate a code blue as soon as possible. The nurse or one of her team members should apply automatic external defibrillator pads in the appropriate positions (the upper right side of the chest and the lower left side of the chest), especially because pulseless ventricular tachycardia is a shockable rhythm. Although nitroglycerin would typically be administered during an MI, it would not be indicated during cardiac arrest. A nonrebreather mask would also not be indicated for a client without a pulse because the client requires bag-valve-mask ventilation per the advanced cardiac life support protocol. The client should be placed in the supine position with a backboard beneath his torso in order for the code team to provide optimal compressions.

5.

- Administer another shock of 200 joules to the client.
- Continue chest compressions at a rate of 120 times per minute.
- Stop the code because the heartbeat has returned to normal.
- Prepare a syringe of 1 mg IV epinephrine.
- Draw blood for laboratory tests: complete blood count, complete metabolic panel, arterial blood gas.

Although the cardiac monitor shows a sinus rhythm, the client still has no pulse, so he is experiencing pulseless electrical activity, which is not a shockable rhythm. The nurse and the code team should continue the code and continue chest compressions at 100–120 beats per minute. During cardiac arrest, epinephrine 1 mg should be administered every 3–5 minutes IV while the client remains pulseless. A member of the code team should also prepare to draw blood for laboratory tests while the code is underway in order to help the team determine the underlying cause of the client's arrest.

6. 1 and 5: Following stent placement, it is essential that the client take an antiplatelet medication, such as clopidogrel, daily for up to 1 year to prevent occlusion of the stent and subsequent MI. The client should also meet with a dietitian, if possible, to learn about the impact of diet on cardiovascular disease. The client should continue to take atorvastatin to lower his cholesterol levels and to prevent further occlusion of the coronary arteries. It is important after an MI to return to exercise as soon as possible—albeit gradually and slowly—to help regain strength, and many clients benefit from specific cardiac rehabilitation programs. The client should be counseled to give up smoking altogether because it increases the likelihood for further cardiac events as well as other diseases.

Standalone Questions

1. 1: Alginate dressings are appropriate for wounds with a large amount of exudate, as they absorb the discharge and form a hydrophilic gel that conforms to the shape of the wound. Because the dressing material (wafers, ropes, fibers) swells in contact with discharge, the wound should be packed loosely. The alginate is covered with a secondary dressing. Hydrocolloid dressings are effective for clean wounds or those with small to moderate exudate. Hydrogel is for dry wounds or those with a small amount of exudate. Transparent film is used with dry wounds.

2. 2: Once a sterile field is contaminated, everything within the field is also considered contaminated, so the nurse must discard the sterile field and gauze pads and start over with new supplies. When establishing a sterile field, the nurse must ensure that the area under the sterile field is clean and dry, as moisture will contaminate the field. The nurse uses clean gloves to remove the old dressing, bare hands or new clean gloves to open the sterile field and gauze packages, and sterile gloves to apply new dressings.

3. 75: In order to complete the calculation, the time needs to be converted to minutes. Three hours and 20 minutes equals 200 minutes. Then, the flow rate (mL per minute) is calculated by dividing the total volume by the minutes:

$$(1{,}000 \text{ mL})/(200 \text{ min}) = 5 \text{ mL/min}$$

Then, the drip rate (drops per minute) is calculated by multiplying the drop factor by the flow rate:

$$(15 \text{ drops/mL}) \times (5 \text{ mL/min}) = 75 \text{ drops/min}$$

4. 1: Loop diuretics, such as furosemide, block chloride and sodium resorption in the ascending limb of the loop of Henle, bringing about rapid diuresis but with major electrolyte disturbance, especially hypokalemia and hyponatremia and to a lesser degree hypocalcemia. Hypokalemia is of most importance because it can result in dysrhythmias with ECG abnormalities, hypotension, lethargy, weakness, nausea and vomiting, paresthesias, muscle cramping, and tetany. Normal values are 3.5–5.5 mEq/L. Potassium supplementation is often given routinely with loop diuretics.

5. 4: The primary risk factor for cervical cancer is a history of human papillomavirus infection. HPV comprises more than 100 viruses. About 40 are sexually transmitted and invade mucosal tissue, causing genital warts (condylomata). An HPV infection causes changes in the mucosa, which can lead to cervical cancer. Over 99% of cervical cancers are caused by HPV, and 70% are related to HPVs 16 and 18. The HPV vaccine, Gardasil, protects against HPVs 6 and 11 (which cause genital warts) and 16 and 18 (which cause cancer). Protection is only conveyed if the female has not yet been infected with these strains.

6. 4: Backward chaining is an approach that teaches the last step in a process first. Once that step is mastered, the next-to-last step is added, and this process continues until the task is mastered. For example, if teaching a child to make a peanut butter and jelly sandwich, the last step would be to place the sandwich on a plate. Therefore, the nurse would do everything leading up to that and then ask the child to put the completed sandwich on the plate, waiting until the child masters this successfully before adding the next-to-the-last step.

7. 4: A client with a severe cough and fever requires both standard precautions and droplet precautions. The best action is to provide the client with a face mask and seat the client in a separate area as far away from other clients as possible to reduce the chance of the infection spreading. A client who is ill should not be sent away or asked to wait outside. The nurse should thoroughly wash his or her hands after contact with the client.

8. 2: Carotemia causes a yellowing of the skin but does not affect the sclera, so the nurse should first ask about the child's diet. Carotemia results from increased levels of beta-carotene in the blood, usually related to high dietary intake of yellow-orange foods, such as sweet potatoes and carrots. Carotemia is common in children if caregivers give the child large amounts of carrots but can also occur in adult vegetarians or people who take excessive carotene nutritional supplements.

9. 4: These symptoms are consistent with mild pacemaker syndrome and occur when the atrial and ventricular contractions are not synchronized properly. This causes decreased cardiac output because the atria do not adequately fill the ventricles. Peripheral vascular resistance increases to compensate initially. Moderate pacemaker syndrome is characterized by increasing dyspnea and orthopnea, dizziness, vertigo, confusion, and sensation of choking. Severe pacemaker syndrome includes pulmonary edema with rales and marked dyspnea, syncope, and heart failure.

10. 2: The AED kit contains cutting shears so that the nurse can quickly expose the chest. The nurse should use the shears to cut away bras with metal wires because the wires may cause arcing during defibrillation. Likewise, any metal piercings on the chest, such as nipple rings, should be removed. The defibrillator electrodes are placed on the right upper chest (negative) and below and lateral to the heart on the left side (positive). AEDs provide spoken messages and diagrams to guide people through the process.

11. 2, 3, 5: Roseola is a contagious disease for which there is no vaccine. It occurs primarily in children between 6 and 24 months of age after the decline of maternal antibodies makes them more susceptible to infection. Roseola is contagious two days before the onset of a fever and is most contagious during the febrile stage, so the child has been exposed to the virus and may still develop the infection, as the incubation period is 9 to 10 days. Roseola is characterized by high fever for 3 to 8 days followed by a pale pink maculopapular rash that lasts 1 to 2 days.

12. 2: Because penicillin may cause an anaphylactic reaction, especially in someone who has previously has a milder reaction, the correct action is to hold the drug and notify the prescribing physician that the client may have had a drug reaction so that the physician can order a skin test or an alternate antibiotic. Common adverse effects of penicillin include a rash, hives, itching, and edema of the face, lips, and/or tongue. Anaphylactic reactions usually occur within 60 minutes of contact with the causative agent.

13. 1: Hypoparathyroidism with hypocalcemia is a complication of thyroidectomy. Hypocalcemia may occur because of inadvertent removal of all or some of the parathyroid glands but may also occur temporarily after surgery because of edema or manipulation of the parathyroid glands during the thyroidectomy. Typical symptoms include a tingling sensation about the mouth and in the fingers and toes. Some may develop severe muscle cramps and tetany. Transient mild hypoparathyroidism may require no treatment, but IV calcium gluconate is indicated for calcium levels below 7 mg/dL.

14. 4: Regardless of experience or position, every nurse is responsible for the safety and welfare of clients, so the nurse should immediately tell the team leader that the irrigating syringe was contaminated and offer to retrieve new sterile supplies. Accidents happen, and one incident does not necessarily mean the team leader is negligent. This is a matter for a supervisor only if the team leader ignores the nurse and continues with the irrigation using a contaminated syringe, putting the client at increased risk of infection.

15. 1: "What aspects of the dying process are you most concerned about?" is the best response because it encourages the client to express her concerns and allows the nurse to assess what can be done to alleviate those concerns. For example, many people facing death are afraid of dying in pain, and the nurse can assure the client that adequate control of pain is almost always possible. This also provides a good opportunity to discuss hospice care. Some clients may express concern about family or financial obligations. These clients may benefit from the assistance of a social worker.

16. 1: The initial intervention when a client reports disturbed sleeping is to complete an assessment of sleep patterns. This should involve questions regarding hours of sleep, quality of sleep, arousals, as well as the number and duration of naps during the day. The client may be asked to keep a sleep diary around the clock, recording sleeping and awakening times, for a few days. Some other initial conservative interventions may include limiting naps and increasing daytime activity, limiting caffeine, maintaining room heat at 70–75 °F, and playing soft soothing music at bedtime.

17. 4: Hypermagnesemia (>2.5 mg/dL) can depress cardiac excitability and conduction, resulting in bradycardia, hypotension, heart block, and the risk of cardiac arrest, depending on the level of magnesium in the blood. Severe hypermagnesemia (>10 mg/dL) is a medical emergency because of the risk of cardiac arrest. Characteristic ECG findings of hypermagnesemia include a flattened P wave, a prolonged PR interval (>0.20 s), a widened QRS complex (>0.12 s), a prolonged QT interval (>0.50 s), and peaked T waves.

18. 1: The most appropriate referral for this client is a speech and language therapist because these professionals are trained to assess dysphagia and provide therapy to improve the ability to swallow. The speech and language therapist may use a number of different strategies to improve swallowing, such as sensory, thermal, suck-swallow, and strengthening exercises, and can provide guidance to staff on compensatory methods to reduce risk of aspiration.

19. 1, 3: The pre-adolescent child needs to be aware of the bodily changes he can expect as he develops secondary sexual characteristics, including normal variations among children and changes in height, weight, and body structure. The mother should allow the child to express changes in the way he thinks and should stress the importance of education. She should also ask the child about issues related to peer pressure, such as bullying, gangs, drugs, tobacco, and alcohol use.

20. 3: Somatic tremor artifacts are the result of involuntary muscle movements, which may occur if the patient is cold and shivering or has a condition that causes tremors, such as Parkinson's disease. Somatic tremor artifacts are characterized by rapid, repetitive, and erratic baseline fluctuations that have no consistent pattern and can be found in all leads; however, they are usually more evident in limb leads. Somatic tremor artifacts may be mistaken for atrial fibrillation.

21. 3: As much as possible, clients with dementia should be oriented to what is true without directly challenging them or telling them they are wrong. The nurse should avoid humoring the client by playing along with her confused statements. In this case, telling the date (July 2) and the time (lunch time) helps to orient the client, and offering to allow the client to watch a movie responds to the client's stated desire to go a movie. If the client becomes extremely agitated at being contradicted, then the best response may be to refocus the client's attention.

22. 1: While protocols may vary slightly, generally those receiving brachytherapy are restricted to a private room during the duration of therapy. Women who are pregnant and children under age 18 may not visit, and visitors are limited to no more than 2 hours visit per day. Visitors must remain at least 6 feet away from the client during visits. Nurses must limit time in the room to that necessary for essential care. Housekeeping staff should be accompanied by a nurse if entering the room is necessary.

23. 4: In ventricular tachycardia (VT), there is reduced cardiac output because the rapid ventricular contractions are inefficient. VT can progress to ventricular fibrillation and cardiac arrest; therefore, VT is an emergent condition. VT is characterized by:

- Rapid ventricular rate (100–250 bpm)
- Absent or dissociated P waves
- Wide QRS complexes (≥0.12 s, or three small boxes)
- Consistent shape and duration of QRS complexes OR changes in shape, amplitude, and direction
- Generally, a regularly spaced RR interval

24. 1, 3: With continuous ambulatory peritoneal dialysis (CAPD) the client instills about 2 liters of fluid over 10–15 minutes and then clamps the tubing. Then, the client folds the tubing and bag over the abdomen and secures it with clothing, maintaining a dwell time of 3 to 5 hours. After this, the tubing is unclamped and dialysate and waste products are drained for about 20 minutes. This drainage is discarded and new dialysate is instilled to begin the cycle again.

25. 2: Generally, the faster the gait, the greater the ambulation speed, the greater expenditure of energy and need for strength. If this 19-year-old client wants to keep pace with his friends and is sufficiently strong and stable, then the fastest gait is the swing-through gait. This gait involves the patient bearing weight on his or her good foot, moving both crutches forward, swinging both legs through and past the crutches, and landing on the good foot. The slowest gait (and the one that requires the least energy) is the 4-point alternate gate.

26. 15: In this case, the calculation involves multiplying the weight in kilograms by the number of milligrams per kilogram: 60 kg × 0.5 mg/kg per 24 hours. Since the drug is to be given in two equal doses (30/2), each dose is 15 mg.

27. 3: While over-medication, delirium, and hypoglycemia may all result in weakness and confusion, when the client was asked to show her teeth, the lips clearly lifted more on the left side than on the right side and more teeth can be observed on the left side. This suggests a weakness or paralysis, consistent with a stroke. Since the weakness is on the right side, the stroke is on the left side. When assessing a stroke patient for facial palsy, the nurse can ask the patient to show her teeth or pantomime the action.

28. 1: First-time mothers, especially, often have little experience with children and are unsure of what to expect. If the mother is concerned that her child cannot crawl at 6 months, then she needs factual information about when to expect the child to crawl, making "Most infants can crawl by 9 months" the best response. The nurse should also assure the mother that infants may vary in their development. A 6-month-old child should be able to sit in tripod position and roll in both directions. Crawling generally follows this, and the child's gross motor skills should improve over the next 3 months.

29. 12: The first calculation is to determine the amount of drug per milligram: 100 mL/10 mg = 10 mg/mL. Then, the total dose is divided by the dose per mL: 120 mg/10 mg per mL = 12 mL. The calculation can also be done by a simple algebraic formula:

$$\frac{100}{10} = \frac{120}{x}$$
$$100x = 1{,}200$$
$$x = 12$$

30. 0.7: The formula for calculating the waist-to-hip ratio is: waist (inches) divided by hips (inches). In this case 28/40 = 0.7. The waist must be measured at its smallest circumference and the hips at the widest. This measurement determines whether a person's body type is classified as "pear" or "apple." People with "apple" shapes have increased abdominal fat, which is a higher health risk than fat in the hips.

Gender	Ideal	Increased risk	High risk
Male	0.9–0.95	0.96–1.0	>1.0
Female	0.7–0.8	0.81–0.85	>0.85

31. 2, 3, 4: This is a sigmoid colostomy, so many of the reabsorptive properties of the colon remain. Because of this, the stool may range from soft to solid. Many clients only expel stool every 2 to 3 days, so the client needs to find what is normal for him. Clients with sigmoid colostomies can often use irrigations to control bowel movements, and some are even able to trigger movements with certain foods or expel stool on a predictable schedule. Clients should be advised of all of the options for appliances and stoma covers.

32. 124: The first step is to convert pounds into kilograms: 136.4 lb/2.2 = 62 kg. Then the total number of kilograms is multiplied by the required grams per kilogram to find the daily total: 62 kg × 2 g/kg = 124 g. Most clients receive 1.5 − 2.0 g/kg/day in TPN solutions.

33. 4: A U wave is a small positive deflection (best observed in leads V2 and V3) that is believed to represent repolarization of the Purkinje fibers, although it is not completely understood. The U wave is most commonly observed in patients with a heart rate of 65 or lower and is generally a normal finding. A prominent U wave can be an indication of hypokalemia or hypercalcemia, but it is also found in healthy athletes. Inverted U waves may be an indication of hypertension or acute ischemia.

34. 1, 3, 4: Motivational interviewing is a nonconfrontational communication approach. Important elements of motivational interviewing include:

- Express empathy instead of criticism.
- Focus on the client's strengths, not weaknesses.
- Avoid confrontation.
- Listen instead of giving advice.
- Recognize that change is the client's responsibility.
- Adjust to resistance from the client rather than oppose.
- Help the client recognize the gap between his or her current situation and goals.

35. 3: Piggyback units should be hung at least 6 inches higher than the primary intravenous unit. Because of the force of gravity when the piggyback unit is infusing, the flow from the primary unit stops until the piggyback unit is empty and then it starts again, so clamping the primary unit tubing is not necessary. During infusion of the piggyback unit, a backcheck valve prevents the piggyback solution from flowing up into the primary unit.

36. 4: Heberden's nodes are characteristic of osteoarthritis. Other findings may include radial deviation of the distal phalanx (fingertip tilted toward the thumb) and Bouchard's nodes (nodules on the proximal interphalangeal joints). Osteoarthritis is usually caused by a previous injury to the joints, so it may occur on one side only, and it is associated with cartilage deterioration. It is slowly progressive with symptoms usually occurring after age 60.

37. 2, 3: During a severe generalized tonic-clonic seizure, the client should be turned to side-lying position to prevent aspiration. Padded tongue blades are no longer utilized with seizures and may cause damage to the mouth and teeth. The side rails should be elevated during the seizure and padded, using pillows or blankets, to prevent a fall from the bed and other injuries. The nurse should not physically restrain a client during a seizure as this may cause injury.

38. 4: Pyridoxine (vitamin B6) can reverse the effects of levodopa in doses exceeding 10 mg. Foods high in vitamin B6 include bran, liver, fish (salmon, cod), pork tenderloin, tahini, molasses, and hazelnuts. Levodopa should be taken with meals to minimize gastrointestinal effects, but these meals should have minimal protein. Clients should eat proteins in small frequent amounts at other times. The client should drink at least 2 liters of fluid daily.

39. 4: The most important point to stress to the client's family about infection control is handwashing. The client and family members should be instructed in proper handwashing technique and the use of alcohol-based hand scrubs. Since a dressing is in place, gowns and gloves are not necessary for all contact with the client. The environmental surfaces should be kept clean.

40. 2: The QRS complex on the ECG tracing shown is approximately 0.32 s (8 small boxes × 0.04 s = 0.32 s). This is an example of ventricular tachycardia (VT) with a wide QRS complex because the QRS complex is greater than 0.12 s (three small boxes). The heart rate is approximately 200 bpm, and P waves and PR intervals are absent. Wide-complex VT may originate in or above the ventricles with abnormal conduction. Wide-complex VT is usually regular.

41. 1, 2, 3, 5: A newly diagnosed client with diabetes type 1 may feel overwhelmed with information, but the nurse must ensure the client understands basic information about glucose testing and insulin administration, skin care, and dietary compliance. The client must also be taught how to respond to signs of hypoglycemia and hyperglycemia and when to call the physician. The client also needs practical information about how to store medications, where to obtain supplies, and how often to have blood tests, such as HbA1c.

42. 3: Fresh frozen plasma replaces plasma but does not contain red blood cells or platelets. It does, however, contain most coagulation factors and complement, so it is the blood product of choice for disorders in which coagulation factors are needed. Whole blood is rarely used but replaces both red blood cells and plasma. Irradiated red blood cells are used to replace red blood cells in those who are immunocompromised. Platelets are used for those with thrombocytopenia.

43. 3: The nurse's initial response should be to express concern to the two (discussing how it is affecting the team) and offer to mediate. The nurse should listen to both sides of the issue and try to help them reach a resolution. If the nurses refuse or the conflict continues, then the nurse should report the situation to the unit supervisor.

44. 3: Even though the client indicated he might want the medication at a later time, the medication must be disposed of following facility protocol with two witnesses, both licensed to dispense medications, who directly observe the disposal and sign a document verifying the disposal. A medication removed from a medicine cart may not be placed back into the cart, and drugs cannot be left at a client's bedside or kept in an unsecure location, such as a tray, for later administration.

45. 1: In this situation, the most appropriate response is to immediately report the incident to a direct supervisor. There should be no attempt at direct confrontation or counsel, as the nurse who took the drug is likely to deny doing so and may become agitated and angry.

46. 4: While consent is usually required for all procedure unless waived by the individual, in an emergency situation when the client's life is at risk and no one is available to sign the consent form, the procedure (in this case for the ruptured spleen) can be carried out. The nurse should immediately transfer the client to the operating room for surgery. In descending order, those who can provide consent if the client is unable to do so include their spouse, adult children, parents, siblings, other relatives, and friends.

47. 3: According to the American Medical Association, informed consent must include the following:

- Explanation of diagnosis
- Nature and reason for treatment or procedure
- Risks and benefits
- Alternative options (regardless of cost or insurance coverage)
- Risks and benefits of alternative options
- Risks and benefits of not having a treatment or procedure

Providing informed consent is a requirement of all states. The client should be given full and clear information prior to signing the consent form and should be encouraged to ask questions to clarify any information that is not clear.

48. 2: Because abusers often accompany victims of domestic abuse to the hospital, the first question should be "Is the person who did this to you present here in the hospital?" If the client answers affirmatively, then security should be called immediately for the client's and nurse's protection. Even if the client answers negatively, the nurse should observe carefully any interactions the client has with someone accompanying her, as she may be too frightened or too ashamed to answer truthfully.

49. 1: Because the onset of symptoms is rapid, these findings are consistent with pulmonary embolism. Acute pulmonary embolism occurs when a thrombus from the venous system or the right side of the heart travels to the lungs and blocks a pulmonary artery or arteriole, resulting in increased alveolar dead space in which ventilation occurs but gas exchange is impaired because of ventilation/perfusion mismatching or intrapulmonary shunting. Common originating sites for thrombus formation are the deep veins in the legs, the pelvic veins, and the right atrium.

50. 1: Hypernatremia results from water deprivation, such as can occur with dehydration, watery diarrhea, burns, diabetes insipidus, heatstroke, and excess sodium chloride administration. Indications include increased serum sodium (>145 mEq/L) but decreased urine sodium, as sodium is reabsorbed by the body rather than excreted through the urine. Urine specific gravity and osmolality are increased because sodium retention results in fluid retention (as the body attempts to compensate) and concentrated urine. Normal value: 135–145 mEq/L; Hyponatremia: <135 mEq/L; Hypernatremia: >145 mEq/L.

51. 150: Current exercise guidelines for adults recommend that they engage in strengthening exercises, such as weight training, twice weekly. They should also engage in aerobic activities of at least 150 minutes per week for moderate activities, such as swimming and walking, or 75 minutes per week for vigorous activities (such as running or aerobic dancing). Clients may be encouraged to join an exercise group or a local gym to encourage compliance.

52. Triage order:

- (First) II. 16-year-old male with a chest injury who is in respiratory distress and severe pain. This patient is first because ABCs are attended to first.
- (Second) IV. Middle-aged male, reeking of alcohol—who is very agitated, hallucinating, and confused—with unknown injuries. This patient is second because he poses a risk to himself and others and may have a head injury or another severe undetected injury.
- (Third) I. 64-year-old female, alert and responsive, with a large laceration of the head. This patient is third because she might have an undetected, underlying head injury.
- (Fourth) III. 28-year-old male with multiple contusions and a fractured right arm. This patient is last because these injuries are not likely to be life-threatening.

53. 3, 4: The nurse should never attempt to push protruding viscera back through an incision. However, the nurse should examine the viscera for indications of ischemia or other tissue damage and cover it with normal saline-soaked dressings to protect the tissue. The client should be placed in low Fowler's position with the head of the bed elevated 15–45 degrees and their knees slightly flexed to reduce tension on the abdominal wound. The client's vital signs must be monitored carefully at least every 15 minutes, and the client must be reassured.

54. 3: If a nurse notes that a portable electrocardiogram machine (or any machine) has a frayed electrical cord, the nurse must immediately remove the machine from service, following established protocols. Because of the danger of fire, neither placing a sign (which may be ignored) on the machine nor leaving the machine and making a report to the unit supervisor would be adequate. The nurse should never place any tape—even electrical tape—around a frayed cord. The cord must be replaced.

55. 2: An infiltration occurs when IV fluid leaks into the surrounding tissue, often causing swelling, discomfort (depending on the solution that has leaked), and cooling of the skin. The cooling of the skin results from the fluid being dispersed in the tissue and is what separates this complication from the others. Sometimes fluid can also be seen leaking from the injection site. In the case of an infiltration, the infusion should be stopped, the IV removed and dressed, the limb elevated, and the registered nurse notified. If the medication being infused is a known irritant, then medications may need to be administered to counteract any damage the solution could do to the tissue.

56. 4: While there is value in all of these approaches—written instructions, help number, questions—the best method is to ask the client to do a return demonstration. This allows the nurse to directly observe and evaluate the client's ability to carry out the needed actions. The client should be able to refer to written directions during the demonstration, but if the client requires the nurse's assistance or becomes confused, this indicates the need for further education.

57. 3: While bedrest alone, with much time in the lateral decubitus position to maximize uterine blood flow, is often indicated for clients with mild preeclampsia, those with severe preeclampsia (BP >160–180/>110 and proteinuria >5 g/24 hours) are usually treated initially with magnesium sulfate (IM or IV) as a prophylaxis to prevent seizures. An antihypertensive, such as hydralazine, is given if the diastolic pressure remains above 110. If seizures (eclampsia) occur, magnesium sulfate or other anticonvulsants, such as diazepam and phenytoin, may be used to prevent recurrence.

58. 20: While the fetal heartbeat may be observed on ultrasound at about 6–7 weeks gestation, it cannot usually be detected by fetoscope until 20 weeks. In early pregnancy, fetal heart tones are often more easily heard above the symphysis pubis, but this position shifts later according to fetal growth and position. Fetal heart tones are more easily detected through the fetus's back, so at later weeks of gestation, the nurse should palpate the fetal position before auscultating.

59. 1: The symptoms are consistent with diabetes mellitus type 1, so the laboratory assessment that is most indicated is blood glucose and HbA1c. The blood glucose level indicates the current level of glucose in the blood (normal value ≤100 mg/dL), but the level may fluctuate throughout the day and vary according to dietary intake. HbA1c provides a more accurate assessment because it shows the average glucose level over a 3-month period. The normal value for HbA1c is <6%.

60. IV, I, II, III: The nurse should prepare the child for the treatment by removing all clothes except the diaper so that as much skin as possible is exposed to the light. The nurse should apply a protective mask over the child's eyes and adjust the light source to 15–20 cm above the child prior to turning on the lights and administering the treatment. Indications include:

Weight	Serum bilirubin level
500–750 g	5–8 mg/dL
751–1000 g	6–10 mg/dL
1001–1250 g	8–10 mg/dL
1251–1500 g	10–12 mg/dL

61. 4: The meal that most corresponds to the dietary guidelines is half of a banana, 1 cup of broccoli, 1 half-cup of quinoa, 3 ounces of roasted turkey, and 8 ounces of 1% milk. The dietary guidelines advise that half of a plate should be filled with fruits and vegetables and that grains should be whole grains (such as quinoa and brown rice). Milk products should be low- or nonfat, and protein should be lean and include limited red meat as well as nonmeat sources of protein, such as beans, eggs, and soy products.

62. 1, 3, 4, 5: Drug compliance is especially important for seizure disorders, and since phenytoin is usually given once or twice daily, the client should establish a routine of taking the drug at the same times each day. Phenytoin may cause gingival hyperplasia, so careful dental care and routine dental evaluations are necessary. Long-term use of phenytoin may also cause osteoporosis, so people should take vitamin D prophylactically, exercise regularly, and have periodic evaluations of osteoporosis to determine if other medications are necessary.

63. 1, 3, 5: The advice that is most important to share with this client is that excessive exposure to the sun increases the risk of skin cancer, and self-tanners are available that do not require sun exposure. Current guidelines suggest that exposing the bare skin for 20 minutes daily is safe and adequate for production of vitamin D. The client should apply sunscreen for exposure of longer duration.

64. 2, 3, 4: The nurse should explain that the immunization cuts the chance of developing shingles in half. Additionally, if the person develops shingles after the immunization, the severity of the infection is usually lessoned and the likelihood of developing postherpetic syndrome, which can result in severe and long-standing pain, is decreased.

65. 3: The most likely reason for the client's response is the placebo effect. The belief that a medication is for pain control can trigger the release of endorphins that, in turn, result in a reduced perception of pain. This does not mean that the pain the client was feeling was imaginary or exaggerated.

66. 1: The initial diagnostic test should be the electrocardiogram because these symptoms are consistent with myocardial infarctions in females, who may not experience the "classic" symptoms of crushing chest pain more associated with males. Females often complain of chest or abdominal tightness and pressure and pain in the neck, jaw, shoulders, or arms rather than the chest. Some clients may complain of "indigestion" and most feel severe fatigue. Nausea, dyspnea, and cold, clammy skin are common findings.

67. 1: When implementing change, the best action to carry out first is to identify and gain support of key staff. In all organizations, there are staff members who are influential for various reasons, and they are usually easy to identify. Once these key staff members (key informants) are on board, they can often influence others to comply.

68. 3: A diet with very little protein will slow the healing process due to a lack of amino acids needed to repair tissue. Clients with wounds need extra protein to promote the healing process, so the client should be carefully assessed by a nutritionist to determine an adequate diet. Usual requirements for healing are 1.25–1.5 g/kg/day of protein.

69. 1: The most therapeutic response would be: "You are worried that you are going to die." Stating in concrete terms what the client is implying gives them the opportunity to discuss their concerns.

70. 3: Junctional escape rhythm occurs when the SA node fails to generate electrical impulses or the impulses are blocked so that the AV node takes over as the pacemaker. This results in retrograde depolarization, which affects the P wave and the PR interval. The P wave and the PR interval are often absent, but the P wave may be inverted or retrograde (after the QRS complex). The heart rate in a junctional escape rhythm is usually 40–60 bpm.

71. 4: The responsibility for ensuring that the task was completed and outcomes were appropriate remains with the delegating nurse, so simply asking if the task was completed is not sufficient. Additionally, the nurse should never assume a task was completed and document accordingly; completion must be verified. When delegating, the nurse should always be mindful of the 5 rights of delegation: right task, right circumstance, right person, right direction, and right supervision.

72. 4: When calculating the duration and amplitude on an ECG, values are typically reported to the nearest 0.5 mm or hundredth of a second if they are slightly above, below, before, or beyond a box unless detailed precision is critical. In this case, the duration of the P wave is 0.12 s (three small boxes, $0.04 \text{ s} \times 3 = 0.12 \text{ s}$), the amplitude is 2 mm (two small boxes, $1 \text{ mm} \times 2 = 2 \text{ mm}$), and the appearance is notched.

73. 2: Because the client has systemic symptoms (fever, chills) and flank pain, these symptoms suggest a kidney infection rather than cystitis. The initial diagnostic tests include a urinalysis and urine culture and sensitivities to determine the causative organism. Clients are usually started on a broad-spectrum antibiotic while awaiting the culture and sensitivity report. In most cases, symptoms recede rapidly once antibiotics are started, so if the infection is severe or the client's condition deteriorates, the client may need hospitalization for intravenous antibiotic therapy.

74. 4: The client is grappling with the spiritual need to forgive. Forgiveness can be very difficult—both forgiving the self and others—and clients may obsess over mistakes they or others have made. Clients may believe that forgiving someone means accepting or condoning the behavior; however, forgiving can be freeing for the client and relieve the stress associated with anger towards someone. Even if clients are unable to forgive, they may be able to make peace with what has occurred and move forward more positively.

75. 2: Methamphetamine is a psychostimulant that can be snorted, ingested orally, smoked, or injected intravenously. While methamphetamine has similar effects to cocaine, the effect is much longer lasting and can persist up to 24 hours. Methamphetamine is often taken with alcohol to temper the anxiety that may occur, but the combination may increase blood pressure and the risk of heart attack or stroke. Methamphetamine users often pick at their skin, leaving lesions that appear as severe acne, and may lose weight because of lack of appetite. "Meth mouth" with dental decay is a common sign.

76. 4: While all of these statements may lead to a discussion about feelings and better management of pain, the statement that suggests a need for education is: "I know all this morphine is making her a drug addict." At one time, healthcare providers withheld pain medication from cancer patients in the mistaken belief that they would become addicts, but the spouse needs to understand the difference between taking narcotics for pleasure and for palliation.

77. 4: When a patient has premature ventricular contractions (PVCs) and ventricular bigeminy, every normal beat is followed by a PVC. PVCs originate from an ectopic focus in the ventricles rather than from the SA node, so there is no P wave before a PVC. PVCs are characterized by a broad QRS complex (≥0.12 s) with abnormal morphology. The PVC occurs earlier than expected. The T wave is negative if the QRS is positive, and it is positive if the QRS is negative.

78. 4: The Unna boot provides support to the calf muscle pump when the client ambulates, so it cannot be used for clients who are not ambulatory. In this case, it should be discontinued until the client is able to resume ambulation. However, it should be replaced with an alternate form of compression, such as compression stockings, to decrease the danger of deep vein thrombosis. Short stretch wrap, such as Comprilan, is also used only with ambulatory clients.

79. 4: Clients are often quite nervous about cardiac monitoring, especially if they are fearful about their condition, and they may dislodge leads so that they can get attention from nurses because they are afraid to be alone or need reassurance. Challenging a client or attempting to make the person feel guilty does not solve the underlying problem. A better approach is for the nurse to take time to talk with the client, explaining how telemetry works, what the numbers and tracings on the monitor mean, and what the staff is learning from the monitoring.

80. 1: The Wong-Baker FACES pain scale is likely the most effective pain scale for assessing pain in a 6-year-old child. FACES can be used for children from about 4 to 16 and also for some adults, especially older adults. FACES comes in both a pediatric and an adult version. Children with normal cognitive ability can usually understand the numeric pain intensity scale by about age 8. The CRIES scale is used for infants, and the PAINAD scale is used for clients with dementia.

81. 1: Pulmonary hygiene is especially important after surgery because inactivity and failure to breathe deeply and cough, aggravated by pain, can result in atelectasis. Patients should be instructed in the use of the incentive spirometer both before surgery and after surgery, and use should be monitored to ensure compliance. Patients with atelectasis typically initially become short of breath and may develop a cough and low-grade fever as secretions pool and the lung collapses. Untreated, the patient may develop hypoxemia, pneumonia, or respiratory failure.

82. 1, 3, 4: If the nurse is discussing the use of a condom, information that is important to share includes:

- Use a condom every time for every sexual encounter.
- Use latex rather than natural membrane condoms for better protection.
- Use only water-based lubricants.
- Use spermicide if trying to prevent pregnancy.
- Hold the condom in place when withdrawing the penis after ejaculation.
- Leave a 1-inch space at the end of the condom to contain ejaculate.

The nurse should also demonstrate how the condom is applied, using a model if one is available.

83. 2: The client's pressure injury is stage II. Wound staging is done according to the following:

- Stage I: Localized intact skin with nonblanchable redness
- Stage II: Partial thickness loss of dermis and red/pink wound surface without slough
- Stage III: Full thickness loss of dermis with subcutaneous tissue exposed. Slough, undermining, and tunneling may be present.
- Stage IV: Full thickness loss of dermis with muscle, tendons, or bones exposed. Slough or eschar may be present.

84. 1, 2, 4: Radiotherapy to the abdominal area and pelvis often damages cells in the intestines, resulting in diarrhea. Clients should be advised to drink 8–12 glasses of clear liquids, eat 5–6 small meals daily, and limit fiber, fat, and lactose (milk products) as they may increase diarrhea. Some people benefit from the BRAT diet (bananas, rice, applesauce, and toast) especially when diarrhea is acute. Clients should also avoid fried and spicy foods, cruciferous vegetables and beans, and soy products.

85. 1, 4: The nurse should advise the client that NSAIDs (e.g., ibuprofen) and salicylates (e.g., aspirin) are OTC anti-inflammatory drugs. Acetaminophen is an antipyretic rather than an anti-inflammatory drug and may help to reduce both pain and fever. Corticosteroids require prescriptions.

86. 1: Women who experience premature rupture of the membranes at term and do not go into labor within 12–24 hours are induced because the risk of infection increases with time. About 9 out of 10 women with premature rupture of the membranes go into labor within 24 hours. In some cases, such as a woman with a history of current or recent vaginal infection or multiple digital vaginal exams, labor may be induced at any time after the membranes rupture.

87. 2, 3: With peripheral arterial insufficiency, the foot exhibits rubor on dependency and pallor on elevation. The skin often feels cool and appears pale and shiny with loss of hair on the leg, foot, and toes. Because of impaired circulation, the toenails may appear thick and ridged. Pedal pulses are weak or absent. Ulcers tend to occur on the tips of toes, between toes, on heels, or on other pressure areas. Ulcers are usually deep, circular, and painful and may be necrotic. Because the venous system may be intact, peripheral edema is usually minimal.

88. 3: The lower border of the blood pressure cuff should be placed at about 2.5 cm above the antecubital crease. The arm should be flexed slightly at the elbow and positioned so that the antecubital crease is at heart level. The inflatable bladder of the cuff should be over the brachial artery. The nurse should palpate the radial pulse while increasing pressure on the cuff, and when the pulse is no longer palpable, raise cuff pressure another 30 mmHg.

89. 3: The WBC and platelet counts are outside normal range:

Test	Result	Normal value
WBC	4.1	4.8-10.8 ($10^3/\mu$L)
RBC	4.38	4.20-5.40 ($10^6/\mu$L)
Hemoglobin	13.8	12.0-16.0 (g/dL)
Hematocrit	42.0	37.0-47.0 (%)
Platelet count	116	150-450 ($10^3/\mu$L)

90. 1: The ECG changes that are seen with both myocardial injury and myocardial infarction include ST-segment elevation and T-wave inversion, so onset of these changes should signal the need for further testing, such as tests for levels of cardiac enzymes and proteins in the blood. In myocardial ischemia, the first stage of heart damage, ST-segment depression, and T-wave inversion are common. In the second stage, when the ischemia is prolonged and damage occurs, ST-segment elevation is evident. In the third stage, myocardial infarction, the first change may be tall T-waves, but these become inverted and ST-segment elevation occurs as the hours pass.

91. 4: ST segment depression occurs when the ST segment is at least 0.5 mm (0.05 mV) below the isoelectric line in ≥2 contiguous leads. The depression may be downsloping, horizontal, or upsloping, depending on the underlying cause. Upsloping ST depression is typically the least concerning. ST segment depression may indicate myocardial ischemia, non-ST elevation myocardial infarction, posterior myocardial infarction, bundle branch block, left ventricular hypertrophy, or electrolyte imbalance, or it may be an effect of digoxin.

92. 1: The blood abnormalities of most concern during treatment of leukemia and most other cancers are thrombocytopenia and neutropenia. About 10% of clients with ALL initially present with disseminated intravascular coagulation (DIC) because of thrombocytopenia. As the platelet level falls, the ability of the blood to clot is impaired and the client is at risk for hemorrhage. The absolute neutrophil count is monitored closely because, as the ANC falls, the risk for exogenous and endogenous infections increases markedly.

93. 2: The client needs to understand the critical importance of using the CPAP machine every time he sleeps. The client's frequent yawning probably indicates that he is not using the machine routinely. Obstructive sleep apnea is characterized by passive collapse of the pharynx during sleep because of upper airway narrowing, often associated with obesity. Patients usually snore loudly with cycles of breath cessation caused by apneic periods lasting up to 60 seconds. These may occur 30 or more times a night despite continued chest wall and abdominal movements, indicating an automatic attempt to breathe.

94. 3: The most appropriate response is to discuss the lack of experience with the unit supervisor, who should adjust the assignment or assign another nurse to assist. The nurse should express a willingness to learn but should be honest about limitations; failing to do so may result in injury to a client.

95. If the nurse must sit a patient who is lying supine in a hospital bed onto the side of the bed in preparation for transfer to a wheelchair, the steps to this procedure are:

1: (First): III. Raise the head of the bed to 30°.
2: (Second) I. Roll the client onto their side, facing the nurse.
3: (Third) II. Place one hand under the shoulders and the other over the hips.
4: (Fourth) IV. Pivot the client into a sitting position.

The nurse must be sure to maintain proper alignment of the client's body and to use correct body mechanics to avoid injuries.

96. 3: While digoxin is used to slow the heart rate, digoxin toxicity may result in either tachycardia or bradycardia as well as almost any type of dysrhythmia. Central nervous system symptoms can include fatigue, headache, and confusion with convulsions with severe toxicity. Clients often complain of GI upsets, including lack of appetite, diarrhea, nausea, and vomiting. They may also report visual disturbances, such as halo vision, colored vision, and flickering lights. The medication should be stopped immediately, cardiac monitoring should be started, and symptoms should be treated as necessary.

97. 3: After administration of a vaginal suppository, the woman must remain in supine position for 5–10 minutes to allow time for the suppository to melt and the medication to spread throughout the vagina. The suppository should be at room temperature prior to administration. If an applicator is available, it should be inserted deeply into the vagina. If inserting the suppository digitally, the finger should be inserted about 2 inches into the vagina so that the suppository rests at the cervix. The woman may want to wear a peri-pad or panty shield to contain any discharge.

98. 3: Infants are usually uncooperative with eye drops and instinctually clinch the eyes tightly to avoid them. The most appropriate method is to gently restrain the head in neutral position while the child is lying supine and place the drops at the inner canthus. When the baby opens the eyes, the fluid will flow into the eye. A caregiver, such as a parent, can assist by restraining the child's head and speaking to the child during the procedure.

99. 1, 2: While most contraceptives are relatively safe for women who smoke, smokers over age 35 are usually advised to avoid combined hormone pills and vaginal rings, such as NuvaRing (which releases both estrogen and progestin). Safer options include progestin-only pills, intrauterine devices, intrauterine systems, diaphragms, implanted contraceptives, and the contraceptive injection.

100. 4: A delta wave appears as a slurring of the upstroke of the QRS complex, which results in a shortened PR interval (<0.12 s) and a widened QRS complex (>0.10 s). This finding is characteristic of Wolff-Parkinson-White syndrome—a congenital cardiac disorder that affects the electrical conduction in the heart. An extra or accessory pathway connects the atria and ventricles, bypassing the AV node. This causes preexcitation of the ventricles and an increased risk of tachyarrhythmias.

Practice Test #2

Case Study 1

The nurse in the emergency department is caring for a 69-year-old male client.

NURSES' NOTES

1115: The client presents to the emergency department reporting shortness of breath (dyspnea), wheezing, and a cough for the past week. He has a barrel-shaped chest on inspection and reports coughing "more often than normal" with increased thick sputum. The client states that he has been using his albuterol inhaler every 3 hours and typically only needs it after moderate exertion. His daughter reports that he has smoked a half a pack of cigarettes per day for the past 46 years and that he usually has dyspnea with moderate exertion but it has progressed to dyspnea at rest within the past week. The client has a history of prostate cancer, hypertension, chronic obstructive pulmonary disease (COPD), and type 2 diabetes mellitus. The client reports that his fasting blood glucose at 0800 today was 104 mg/dL. On assessment, the client is experiencing dyspnea when answering questions and is only able to speak a few words at a time. The client's daughter states that he has appeared to be increasingly anxious over the past 3 days. His skin is warm and dry, and inspiratory and expiratory wheezing is auscultated bilaterally.

VITAL SIGNS

	1115
Temp	98.4 °F axillary
HR	102, irregular
BP	184/74
RR	23
Pulse oximetry	86% on room air

1. From the following list, select the assessment findings that require <u>immediate</u> follow-up. (Select all that apply)

1. Fasting blood glucose
2. Dyspnea and cough
3. Pulse oximetry reading
4. Anxiety
5. Barrel-shaped chest
6. Pulse, respirations, and blood pressure
7. Warm, dry skin
8. Medical history

2. Based on the client's current clinical picture, he is at the <u>highest</u> risk for developing

_____.

1. respiratory alkalosis
2. respiratory acidosis
3. diabetic ketoacidosis
4. metabolic acidosis

NURSES' NOTES

1130: The client is sitting in a tripod position with increased work of breathing. His pulse oximetry reading is 83% on room air. The client states "I can't catch my breath," pausing to take a breath between each word. The client is less responsive to questions and appears tired. The primary physician was notified, and new orders are being placed.

VITAL SIGNS

	1115	1130
Temp	98.4 °F axillary	98.4 °F axillary
HR	102, irregular	104, irregular
BP	184/74	180/74
RR	23	27
Pulse oximetry	86% on room air	83% on room air

3. The nurse receives the following orders. Highlight all orders from the following list that the nurse should consider a <u>priority</u>.

- Administer oxygen, 4 L/min via nasal cannula.
- Chest x-ray.
- Administer albuterol nebulization treatment.
- Collect samples for laboratory tests: sputum culture, complete blood count (CBC), and arterial blood gas (ABG).

NURSES' NOTES

1200: The client's ABGs are taken at the bedside by the respiratory therapist, and the physician is notified of the results.

LABORATORY RESULTS

Laboratory Test and Reference Range	Result
pH Adult: 7.35–7.45	7.32
PaO$_2$ Adult: >90 mmHg	58
PaCO$_2$ Adult: 35–45 mmHg	48
HCO^3 Adult: 18–24 mEq/L	25

4. Based on the results of the arterial blood gases collected bedside, the nurse anticipates interventions to address the client's _____ using _____.

Blank 1:

1. compensated respiratory alkalosis
2. uncompensated respiratory alkalosis
3. compensated respiratory acidosis
4. uncompensated respiratory acidosis

Blank 2:

1. mechanical ventilation
2. BiPAP
3. increased oxygen via nasal cannula
4. extracorporeal membrane oxygenation

5. For the following list of potential nursing interventions, specify whether each one is indicated or not indicated.

Potential Nursing Interventions	Indicated	Not Indicated
Anticipate an order for a Foley catheter.	O	O
Assist the client into a supine position.	O	O
Apply a bordered foam dressing to protect the client's skin.	O	O
Educate the patient and family on the reason for using BiPAP.	O	O
Monitor the patient for abdominal distension.	O	O

NURSES' NOTES

1300: The client is resting in his room, interacting appropriately with his daughter. Repeat ABGs are taken at the bedside by a respiratory therapist. The client is able to answer assessment questions in short sentences and denies anxiety, pain, and discomfort at this time.

VITAL SIGNS

	1115	1130	1300
Temp	98.4 °F axillary	98.4 °F axillary	98.5 °F axillary
HR	102, irregular	104, irregular	121, irregular
BP	184/74	180/74	172/80
RR	23	27	19
Pulse oximetry	86% on room air	83% on room air	92% on BiPAP

LABORATORY RESULTS

Laboratory Test and Reference Range	Result
pH Adult: 7.35–7.45	7.37
PaO$_2$ Adult: >90 mmHg	82
PaCO$_2$ Adult: 35–45 mmHg	43
HCO^3 Adult: 18–24 mEq/L	23

6. The client has been reevaluated to determine his response to the initial interventions provided. Of the following list of assessment findings, specify whether each one indicates that the client's condition has improved, is unchanged, or has worsened.

Assessment Findings	Improved	Unchanged	Worsened
Dyspnea while talking	O	O	O
Respirations, 19	O	O	O
Temperature, 98.5 °F axillary	O	O	O
Pulse oximetry reading, 92%	O	O	O
Heart rate, 121 and irregular	O	O	O
pH, 7.37	O	O	O
PaCO$_2$, 43	O	O	O

Case Study 2

A 19-year-old male arrives to the emergency department via ambulance.

NURSES' NOTES

1900: A 19-year-old male client arrives to the emergency department via ambulance clutching at the left side of his chest, visibly struggling to breathe, and appearing anxious. The client reports that he was watching television with his family when he felt a sudden sharp pain (rated 10/10) to his left chest and could not catch his breath. The client denies any recent trauma or illness. The client appears to be tall and relatively thin for his age. The client denies any known medical history, is not taking any medications, and is up to date on his vaccines. Emergency medical services (EMS) did a preliminary 12-lead electrocardiogram (EKG), which showed that the client was in sinus tachycardia. EMS also reports administering an albuterol nebulizer en route to the hospital with no relief to the client. The client is placed on cardiac monitoring, an IV access is established, and a set of vital sign measurements is obtained.

VITAL SIGNS

	1900
Temp	97.7 °F temporal
HR	115
BP	105/86
RR	35
Pulse oximetry	92% on room air

PHYSICAL ASSESSMENT

Body System	1900
Neurological	The client is alert and oriented ×4. There are no neurological deficits noted.
Pulmonary	The client's breathing is labored and tachypneic. He appears to be using his accessory muscles. Lung sounds are absent on the left side. His trachea is midline.
Cardiovascular	The cardiac monitor shows that the client is in sinus tachycardia. His pulses are strong. No jugular vein distension is noted.
Integumentary	Skin appears pale with cyanosis developing in the lips.

1. From the following list, select the assessment findings that require <u>immediate</u> follow-up. (Select all that apply)

1. EKG findings
2. Respiratory rate
3. Integumentary assessment
4. Height and weight
5. Work of breathing
6. Lung sounds

2. Based on the nurse's assessment findings, the nurse should recognize that the client is <u>most</u> likely experiencing a(n) _____.

1. myocardial infarction
2. anxiety attack
3. asthma exacerbation
4. spontaneous pneumothorax
5. tension pneumothorax

3. The nurse receives the following orders. Highlight all orders from the following list that the nurse should consider a <u>priority</u>.

- Obtain a chest x-ray.
- Obtain an arterial blood gas (ABG) reading.
- Administer supplemental oxygen.
- Administer IV morphine.
- Start a second large-bore IV.
- Obtain a repeat EKG.

NURSES' NOTES

1920: The client is place on supplemental oxygen via a simple mask. The repeat EKG continues to show that the client is in sinus tachycardia. A chest x-ray is obtained and shows pneumothorax to the left lung. ABGs are normal. The nurse places a second IV and administers IV morphine. The client reports that he is now in 8/10 pain, but that he continues to struggle to breathe.

4. For the following list of potential nursing interventions, specify whether each one is indicated or not indicated.

Potential Nursing Interventions	Indicated	Not Indicated
Prepare to intubate.	○	○
Prepare the client for the cardiac catheterization lab.	○	○
Prepare for chest tube placement.	○	○
Request an order for further analgesia.	○	○
Prepare for cardioversion.	○	○

NURSES' NOTES

1945: The health care team prepares for chest tube placement. The nurse sets up the chest tube system and administers IV fentanyl. The physician administers local anesthesia and places a chest tube. The client reports that his pain is now 3/10 and he immediately stops using his accessory muscles when breathing. The blue tint leaves the client's lips. Maintaining sterile technique, the nurse and physician hook the chest tube up to the system.

	1900	1945
Temp	97.7 °F temporal	98.1 °F temporal
HR	115	95
BP	105/86	90/76
RR	35	22
Pulse oximetry	92% on room air	95% on room air

5. For the following list of assessment findings, specify whether each one indicates that the client's condition has improved, is unchanged, or has worsened.

Assessment Findings	Improved	Unchanged	Worsened
Pain, 3/10	○	○	○
Respirations, 22	○	○	○
Blood pressure, 90/76	○	○	○
Pulse oximetry, 95%	○	○	○
Integumentary assessment	○	○	○

6. The client has orders for admission to the floor. In caring for a client with a chest tube for a pneumothorax, which of the following findings are <u>expected</u>? (Select all that apply)

1. Rise and fall of the water seal in the chest tube system with client breathing
2. Increased work of breathing
3. Decreased work of breathing
4. Blood drainage in the atrium
5. Continuous bubbling in the water seal
6. A change in depth of the chest tube with client ambulation

Case Study 3

A 65-year-old female arrives to the emergency department via ambulance.

NURSES' NOTES

1600: A 65-year-old female client is brought into the emergency department via ambulance. The client reports that she called 911 after she had trouble getting out of bed that morning. She also states that she has been nauseous, complaining of generalized abdominal pain and chest pain since that morning. The client has a history of renal failure, hypertension, and diabetes mellites type 2. The client reports that she is on dialysis and that she had missed her appointment the day before. Emergency medical services (EMS) ran a 12-lead electrocardiogram (EKG) that revealed peaked T-waves. EMS also administered 324 mg aspirin to the client prior to her arrival at the hospital. The client is changed into a gown and placed on the cardiac monitor, an IV is started, labs are drawn, and vital sign measurements are taken.

VITAL SIGNS

	1600
Temp	97.5°F temporal
HR	68
BP	185/95
RR	16
Pulse oximetry	96% on room air

PHYSICAL ASSESSMENT

Body System	**1600**
Neurological	The client is alert and oriented ×4. She is complaining of generalized weakness and an inability to get out of bed.
Pulmonary	The client's breath sounds are clear. Her breathing pattern is regular.
Cardiovascular	The client is complaining of chest pain. Her EKG shows peaked T-waves within what is otherwise a sinus rhythm. Also, +1 edema is noted to the bilateral lower extremities.
Integumentary	A fistula is noted on the left forearm. Her skin is otherwise normal in appearance.
Gastrointestinal	The client is complaining of nausea. Her abdomen is cramping throughout, but it is nontender.

LABORATORY RESULTS

Laboratory Test and Reference Range	**1600**
Red blood cell (RBC) count Adult female: 4.5–5.0 ×10^6/mm³	4.7
White blood cell (WBC) count Adult/child >2 years: 5,000–10,000/mm³	9,000
Glucose Adult: 70–110 mg/dL	235
Troponin Adult: <0.4 ng/mL	0.00
Potassium Adult: 3.5–5.0 mmol/L	7.0
Creatinine 0.7–1.3 mg/dL	8.5

1. From the following list, select the assessment findings that require <u>immediate</u> follow-up. (Select all that apply)

1. Missed dialysis appointment
2. Serum glucose
3. Serum creatinine
4. Serum potassium
5. Blood pressure
6. Troponin

2. If left untreated, the client is <u>most</u> at risk of developing _____.

1. myocardial infarction
2. diabetic ketoacidosis
3. congestive heart failure
4. cardiac arrhythmia

3. The nurse receives the following orders. Highlight all orders from the following list that the nurse should consider a <u>priority</u>.

- Obtain a computed tomography (CT) scan of the abdomen with contrast.
- Administer IV dextrose and insulin.
- Administer IV calcium.
- Administer IV ondansetron.
- Obtain a chest x-ray.

NURSES' NOTES

1630: The nurse administers IV dextrose and insulin. The nurse then starts the IV calcium drip. A chest x-ray is obtained and shows no signs of pulmonary edema or cardiomegaly.

4. For the following list of potential nursing interventions, specify whether each is indicated or not indicated.

Potential Nursing Interventions	Indicated	Not Indicated
Request an order for a fluid bolus.	O	O
Request an order for a repeat basic metabolic panel.	O	O
Recheck at the bedside the serum glucose.	O	O
Start a second IV in the left arm.	O	O
Provide continuous cardiac monitoring.	O	O

NURSES' NOTES

1730: The client requests to walk to the bathroom. The client is steady on her feet without staff assistance. The client also states that her nausea has decreased and she would like to eat whenever able.

	1600	1730
Temp	97.5°F temporal	98.5°F temporal
HR	68	70
BP	185/95	175/80
RR	16	18
Pulse oximetry	96% on room air	97% on room air

LABORATORY RESULTS

Laboratory Test and Reference Range	1600	1730
Glucose Adult: 70–110 mg/dL	235	75
Troponin Adult: <0.4 ng/mL	0.00	0.01
Potassium Adult: 3.5–5.0 mmol/L	7.0	5.2
Creatinine 0.7–1.3 mg/dL	8.5	8.4

5. For the following list of assessment findings, specify whether each one indicates that the client's condition has improved, is unchanged, or has worsened.

Assessment Findings	Improved	Unchanged	Worsened
Glucose, 75	O	O	O
Troponin, 0.01	O	O	O
Potassium, 5.2	O	O	O
Client's neurological assessment	O	O	O
Client's gastrointestinal assessment	O	O	O

6. The client is being admitted to the floor. The nurse anticipates that the plan of care will include _____, _____, and _____. (Select three answers)

    1. dialysis
    2. telemetry monitoring
    3. a continuous insulin drip
    4. IV furosemide
    5. repeat serum potassium labs

Standalone Questions

1. A patient is admitted with presumed appendicitis. In which abdominal quadrant should the nurse anticipate the patient to be experiencing the most pain?

1. RUQ
2. LUQ
3. RLQ
4. LLQ

2. A client with uterine cancer is receiving intracavity irradiation with an intrauterine "stem" device. On examination, the nurse discovers that the radiation source has become dislodged and is partially outside of the vagina. Which action should the nurse carry out?

1. Wear rubber gloves to lift the stem and place it in a shielded container.
2. Immediately notify the radiation department.
3. Cover the stem with a folded towel to protect the client's skin.
4. Use rubber gloves to gently reinsert the stem into the vagina.

3. Which of the following is an indication of primary graft dysfunction in a lung transplant recipient?

1. Frequent oxygen desaturation
2. Chest pressure
3. Fever
4. Cough

4. A pregnant woman admitted for preeclampsia experiences a seizure. In what position should the nurse place the client during the seizure?

1. Supine semi-Fowler's position
2. Right lateral
3. Supine flat position
4. Left lateral

5. The most common route of entry of microbial agents into the lungs is through:

1. Aspiration
2. Translocation from the GI tract
3. Inhalation
4. Vascular spread from a distant site

6. When the nurse enters the break room, she finds that a colleague is sharing personal information about his client with other staff members. What is the best action for the nurse?

1. Leave the break room.
2. Report the situation to a supervisor.
3. Tell the colleague that he should not be talking about a client.
4. Tell the colleague and staff members that she is not comfortable violating a client's privacy.

7. A train accident has resulted in many severe casualties, and the emergency department is inundated with clients, but few hospital beds are available. What is the best solution to this emergency situation?

1. Transfer incoming clients to other facilities as soon as they are stabilized.
2. Place newly admitted clients in the hallways.
3. Close the emergency room to further clients.
4. Carry out early discharge for low-risk, noncritical clients to free up some beds.

8. The nurse is caring for a three-year-old child with sickle cell anemia. The nurse expects that the child will receive which of the following treatments routinely as prophylaxis to prevent complications? *Select all that apply.*

1. Penicillin
2. Blood transfusions
3. Hydroxyurea
4. Opioids
5. Oxygen therapy

9. When educating parents on the dangers of choking, the nurse should advise that children under 3 years of age should not be fed which of the following foods? *Select all that apply.*

1. Beef
2. Peanuts
3. Popcorn
4. Round hard candies
5. Hot dogs
6. Cooked carrots

10. A 16-year-old female client is hospitalized for anorexia nervosa. Which of the following behaviors should the nurse report to the physician? *Select all that apply.*

1. The client walks about the grounds with her friend each morning.
2. The client jogs in place for extended periods of time three or four times daily.
3. The client complains daily about constipation, demanding laxatives.
4. The client drinks one to two liters of water daily.
5. The client states that she doesn't need to be in the hospital and refuses to leave her room or interact with other clients.

11. The nurse is irrigating a Foley urinary catheter using open intermittent irrigation and has instilled 30 mL of fluid, but the fluid does not drain back after the syringe is removed. What is the next step the nurse should carry out?

1. Turn the client onto the side facing the nurse.
2. Notify the physician.
3. Aspirate the fluid with the syringe.
4. Instill another 30 mL of fluid and then check for drainage.

12. A client is undergoing negative pressure wound therapy (NPWT). Which of the following tasks associated with NPWT can be delegated to unlicensed assistive personnel (UAP)? *Select all that apply.*

1. Disconnect the NPWT unit and remove dressings.
2. Apply new dressings and connect the NPWT unit.
3. Report changes in the client's comfort level.
4. Monitor tubing to prevent displacement when turning the client.
5. Assess the condition of the wound.

13. The physician has written an order for the nurse to remove a client's running sutures since the incision is well healed. The running suture line has 8 stitches (including the knotted stitches at the ends). When the suture removal is completed, how many individual pieces of suture should the nurse have removed?

1. One
2. Two
3. Three
4. Eight

14. A client receiving packed red blood cells complains of itching and is developing hives and local erythema around the IV insertion site.

I. Notify the physician.
II. Stop the transfusion.
III. Notify the blood bank.
IV. Administer medications as ordered.

Place the actions (in Roman numerals) in the correct order from the first to the last.

1. _____
2. _____
3. _____
4. _____

15. A 90-year-old client with moderate Alzheimer's disease lives with her son and daughter-in-law. Which statement by the daughter-in-law suggests a need for more education about the disease?

1. "She purposely hides her belongings from me."
2. "I have to keep the doors latched at all times."
3. "She thinks I'm her mother at times."
4. "She can't remember where the bathroom is located."

65

16. A 66-year-old monogamous male with low risk factors states that he has not had a physical examination or any medical care for 15 years and asks the nurse if he needs immunizations. Which of the following immunizations should the nurse recommend? *Select all that apply.*

1. Influenza vaccination
2. Pneumococcal vaccination
3. Tetanus-diphtheria booster
4. Herpes zoster (shingles) vaccination
5. Human papillomavirus (HPV) vaccination
6. Mumps, measles, rubella (MMR) vaccination

17. A client has been prescribed 96 mg of theophylline, which is available as 80 mg per 15 mL. How many mL should the client receive? *Record your answer as a whole number.*

_____ mL

18. A client receiving total parenteral nutrition (TPN) is exhibiting lethargy, changes in mental status, and asterixis (flapping tremors of the hands). Which of the following interventions should the nurse anticipate?

1. Increase the dextrose concentration of the formula.
2. Decrease the dextrose concentration of the formula.
3. Decrease the protein concentration of the formula.
4. Increase lipid intake.

19. A client receiving radiation to the abdomen complains of almost-constant diarrhea. Which of the following should the client do to manage diarrhea? *Select all that apply.*

1. Drink eight or more cups of clear liquids daily.
2. Increase intake of high-fiber foods.
3. Drink three to four cups of milk daily.
4. Eat five to six small meals daily.
5. Take Imodium as prescribed.
6. Use baby wipes to cleanse the rectal area.

20. Although the sister of a client with end-stage kidney disease has stated she will donate a kidney to her brother, she actually does not want to do so even though testing shows she is a good match. However, she does not want her brother or family to know that she has refused to donate a kidney. If the client asks if his sister is being honest about not being a match, which of the following is the most appropriate response?

1. "I don't believe she was a match."
2. "You should ask your sister."
3. "I don't know the answer to that question."
4. "You should discuss that with your doctor."

21. Which of the following is the most effective method for reducing the spread of nosocomial infections, such as *C.lostridioides difficile?*

1. Placing clients in private rooms
2. Providing antibiotic prophylaxis
3. Cleaning the rooms with a disinfectant
4. Practicing a thorough and consistent handwashing routine

22. A patient underwent a fiberoptic bronchoscopy for a right lung biopsy under conscious sedation. Within a few minutes of being sent to the recovery room, the client shows increasing signs of dyspnea and, although groggy, has ipsilateral chest pain. The pulse rate increases from 82 to 100, and the client is slightly hypotensive and coughing. Which of the following should the nurse suspect?

1. Heart attack
2. Pulmonary edema
3. Pneumothorax or bleeding
4. Pulmonary embolism

23. When the nurse is doing a physical exam, which part of the hand is most sensitive to temperature variations?

1. The thumb
2. The fingertips
3. The palm
4. The dorsum

24. When conducting a physical exam and assessing the apical pulse in an adult client, where should the nurse place the stethoscope?

1. Second left intercostal space at the midclavicular line
2. Fourth left intercostal space at the sternal margin
3. Fourth left intercostal space at the midclavicular line
4. Fifth left intercostal space at the midclavicular line

25. A 52-year-old client tells the nurse that her yearly Pap smears have always been negative, and she asks if she needs continue to have a Pap smear yearly. Which of the following is the best recommendation?

1. "You should continue with yearly Pap smears."
2. "You should have Pap smears every two to three years."
3. "You should have Pap smears every five years."
4. "You no longer need to have Pap smears."

26. A client arrives at the emergency department with a sliver of metal penetrating his right eye, resulting from a work injury. Which of the following initial actions should the nurse anticipate?

1. Cover the affected eye with a patch.
2. Irrigate the affected eye.
3. Remove the penetrating object with forceps.
4. Request a consultation with an ophthalmologist.

27. The Tensilon (edrophonium chloride) test is used to diagnose which of the following?

1. Myasthenia gravis
2. Multiple sclerosis
3. Parkinson's disease
4. Bell's palsy

28. In many cultures, pregnancy is viewed as a natural condition rather than a medical condition. How does this affect prenatal care?

1. Pregnant women often seek prenatal care later and less frequently.
2. These views have little effect on prenatal care.
3. Pregnant women believe prenatal care is harmful to the fetus.
4. These views often result in increased rates of fetal mortality.

29. A client who has been taking oral prednisone to control his chronic obstructive pulmonary disease (COPD) wants to transition to inhaled corticosteroids. The nurse anticipates which of the following scenarios?

1. The client must be tapered from the oral drug while beginning treatment with the inhaled drug.
2. The client must be tapered from the oral drug before beginning treatment with the inhaled drug.
3. The oral medication can be discontinued immediately, and the client can be started on the inhaled drug.
4. The oral medication cannot be discontinued, so the client cannot transition to the inhaled drug.

30. Which of the following findings place a client at a high risk for suicide? *Select all that apply.*

1. Older age
2. A previous violent suicide attempt (using a knife or gun)
3. A previous suicide attempt at an isolated site
4. A history of depression 10 years previously
5. A current history of mental illness and disordered thinking

31. A client has had a ventricular pacemaker implanted, but he is experiencing lethargy, headache, pain in the jaw, breathlessness, and anxiety. On examination, the nurse notes pulsations evident in the neck and the abdomen. Which of the following is the most likely reason for the client's symptoms?

1. The client is having a panic attack.
2. The client is experiencing pacemaker syndrome.
3. The client is having a myocardial infarction.
4. The client is experiencing pacemaker-mediated tachycardia.

32. A 76-year-old client became a widow 10 years previously, but she speaks about her husband almost constantly, visits his grave daily, cries daily, and appears unable to make decisions or care for herself because of grief. How would the nurse best describe the client's grieving?

1. Prolonged
2. Normal
3. Delayed
4. Distorted

33. A client with ovarian cancer works for a small company with six employees and asks the nurse if she is allowed accommodations at work because of her cancer under provisions of the Americans with Disabilities Act (ADA). Which is the best response?

1. "The company must accommodate your needs under provisions of the ADA."
2. "The company is exempt from the provisions of the ADA because of its size."
3. "The company must allow you time for treatment but can require you to continue to work full time."
4. "Cancer is not considered a disability, so the provisions of the ADA do not apply."

34. Under which delivery care model would the nurse expect to be responsible for the least number of clients?

1. Functional
2. Total patient care
3. Team nursing
4. Modified primary care

35. A client with Alzheimer's disease is hospitalized after a mild stroke. The client calls out frequently and often tries to climb out of bed. What is the best room assignment for the client?

1. A private room within the line of sight of the nursing station
2. A private room at the end of the hallway away from other, more critically ill, clients
3. A shared room with another cognitively impaired client
4. Any room as long as the client is physically restrained

36. Following a stroke, a client has impaired swallowing and is unable to feed himself. What is the best position to place the client in when preparing to assist him with meals?

1. Semi-Fowler's position with head in midline and chin tilted upward
2. Supine position with head in midline and chin tilted downward
3. Upright position with head in midline and chin tilted downward
4. Upright position with head in midline and chin tilted upward

37. If monitoring a client's control of diabetes, which of the following sources of information is the most reliable?

1. Serum glucose level
2. HbA1c
3. Client's food and exercise log
4. Client's prescribed diet

38. According to federal law, if a client dies in a hospital setting, which of the following must be done by the staff?

1. The coroner must be notified.
2. The family decision maker must be asked about organ donation.
3. The family must be provided information about funeral regulations.
4. The Social Security Administration must be notified.

39. A 58-year-old client is to be discharged after hip replacement surgery. What adaptive equipment does the nurse expect that the client will need initially in the home? *Select all that apply.*

1. A walker
2. An elevated toilet seat
3. A wheelchair
4. A reacher/grabber
5. A sock aid

40. The nurse is caring for a dying client. Which of the following symptoms indicate that death will occur within a few days? *Select all that apply.*

1. The client is increasingly lethargic and disoriented.
2. The client has increasing dysphagia.
3. The client is extremely weak, gaunt, and pale.
4. The client is drinking only four or five ounces of water at a time.
5. The client is incontinent of a small amount of concentrated urine.
6. The client has a decreased cardiac rate.

41. A client with moderately advanced dementia is frequently incontinent of urine. Which scheduled urination regimen is most appropriate for this client?

1. Bladder training
2. Timed voiding
3. Patterned urge response toileting
4. Prompted voiding

42. A client is treated in the emergency department for rape, and a rape kit is completed. The client remains calm, staring at the wall, and she does not appear upset or traumatized, stating repeatedly that she is "fine." Based on these observations, the nurse believes which of the following?

1. The client is in a state of denial.
2. The client is lying about the rape.
3. The client is in shock.
4. The client suffered a head injury during the rape.

43. Which of the following descriptions fit the profile of an infant abductor? *Select all that apply.*

1. Female, approximately age 30
2. Male, approximately age 30
3. A frequent visitor to the nursery
4. A visitor who asks many questions about nursery and hospital procedures
5. A frequent, friendly visitor who chats with staff and parents, getting to know them
6. A person with a criminal record

44. A client has been admitted to the mental health unit for bipolar disorder. On the care plan, the nurse has listed "chronic low self-esteem" as a nursing diagnosis with "self-esteem enhancement" and "self-awareness enhancement" as interventions. Which of the following would the nurse include as expected outcomes? *Select all that apply.*

1. The client is able to use positive self-talk to interrupt negative thinking.
2. The client is able to develop strategies to increase his interactions with others.
3. The client is able to verbalize the symptoms of bipolar disorder and the treatments.
4. The client is able to use positive coping behaviors to improve his functioning.
5. The client is able to develop satisfying personal relationships.

45. A client receiving oral tetracycline for the treatment of acne should be advised to avoid which of the following?

1. Sunbathing
2. Swimming
3. Running
4. Weight lifting

46. Which of the following drugs is the appropriate antidote for an overdose of acetaminophen?

1. Protamine sulfate
2. Folic acid
3. Naloxone
4. *N*-acetylcysteine

47. The client is to use a metered-dose inhaler (MDI) without a spacer for albuterol. How should the nurse advise the client to position the inhaler for self-administration?

1. In her mouth with her lips sealed around the opening
2. Touching her lips but outside of the mouth
3. One to two inches in front of her mouth
4. Three to four inches in front of her mouth

48. A client with extensive burns of the lower extremities is treated with topical agents, and the burns are wrapped with several layers of dressings. On examination, the nurse finds that the peripheral pulses are diminished. Which is the best initial action for the nurse?

1. Elevate the extremities to reduce edema.
2. Remove the dressings.
3. Loosen the dressings.
4. Reevaluate the peripheral pulses after 15 minutes.

49. A 48-year-old female client complains of episodes of severe right upper quadrant abdominal pain lasting two to six hours, indigestion, nausea and vomiting, and clay-colored stools. The nurse suspects the client may have which of the following diagnoses?

1. Colitis
2. Pancreatitis
3. Cholecystitis
4. Diverticulitis

50. The physician has ordered wrist restraints for a client who is confused, combative, and attempting to pull out her Foley catheter. Which of the following actions can the nurse delegate to unlicensed assistive personnel? *Select all that apply.*

1. Application of restraints
2. Assessing the continued need for restraints
3. Reviewing the correct placement of restraints
4. Repositioning the client while in restraints
5. Decision regarding the type of restraints needed

51. If a client is to undergo gastric lavage after ingesting poison, what position should the nurse place the client in for the procedure?

1. Semi-Fowler's position with head elevated to 30–40 degrees
2. Upright position with head elevated to 80–90 degrees
3. Trendelenburg position with the client supine
4. Left lateral position with head lowered 15 degrees

52. A client tells the nurse, "I was awake half the night suffering!" Which of the following responses demonstrates therapeutic communication?

1. "Your pain is not well controlled."
2. "You should have asked for more pain medication."
3. "Why didn't you call the nurse?"
4. "You poor thing. I'm so sorry."

53. The nurse is caring for a client who is undergoing peritoneal dialysis. How long does the nurse expect that a typical exchange cycle (infusion, dwell time, and drainage) will take to complete?

1. 12 hours
2. 3–4 hours
3. 60–90 minutes
4. 30–45 minutes

54. Which of the following positions may result in blood pooling in the extremities, decreased blood pressure (BP) and cardiac output, increased respiratory effort, decreased lung compliance, and decreased cerebral circulation?

1. Trendelenburg
2. Right side-lying
3. Supine
4. Prone

55. Which of the following interventions are indicated as part of post-mortem care? *Select all that apply.*

1. Position the body with limbs in proper alignment.
2. Dress the client in burial clothing.
3. Place dentures in the mouth.
4. Cleanse the body gently as necessary.
5. Tape the eyes closed or place weighted items on the eyelids.

56. A client with severe diarrhea, nausea, and vomiting has become increasingly lethargic and weak with tingling in the hands and feet, muscle cramps and tetany, hypotension, and dysrhythmias with ECG abnormalities that include PVCs and flattened T waves. Based on these signs and symptoms, which of the following electrolyte imbalances should the nurse suspect?

1. Hypokalemia
2. Hyperkalemia
3. Hyponatremia
4. Hypernatremia

57. If a patient was involved in a motorcycle accident and is unresponsive and on a ventilator, which of the following tests must be performed to diagnose brain death prior to organ donation? *Select all that apply.*

1. Two electroencephalograms (EEGs) taken 12–24 hours apart
2. Two electrocardiograms (ECGs) taken 12–24 hours apart
3. Testing of brainstem reflexes
4. Apnea testing
5. Transcranial Doppler ultrasonography

58. A client with chronic obstructive pulmonary disease (COPD) feels breathless despite oxygen administration and bronchodilators. Which of the following positions should the nurse place the client in to best relieve breathlessness?

1. Semi-Fowler's, at 30°
2. High Fowler's, upright at 90°
3. Semi-Fowler's, at 45°
4. Leaning forward at 30–40°

59. A child weighing 30 kg is being treated with Zosyn (piperacillin/tazobactam) IV every eight hours with a dose of 100 mg piperacillin/12.5 mg tazobactam per kg of body weight. What is the child's correct dosage in grams (g)?

1. 3,000 g piperacillin/375 g tazobactam
2. 30 g piperacillin/37.5 g tazobactam
3. 3 g piperacillin/3.75 g tazobactam
4. 3 g piperacillin/0.375 g tazobactam

60. Which of the following are HIPAA violations? *Select all that apply.*

1. The nurse shares information about the client with the client's sister.
2. The nurse allows another nurse to "shoulder surf" the client's HER.
3. The nurse accesses the history and physical of a client assigned to the nurse.
4. The nurse discusses the client's concerns about treatment with the physician.
5. The nurse tells the client's physician that the client expressed suicidal ideation.

61. The nurse believes that the dosage of a medication is too high for a client, based on the recommended mg per kg of weight. Which of the following initial actions should the nurse carry out?

1. Contact the pharmacy to determine if the dosage is within acceptable limits.
2. Notify the supervisor of her concerns.
3. Telephone the physician to question the dosage.
4. Assume the dosage was verified when ordered, and administer the drug.

62. What does the following ECG strip represent?

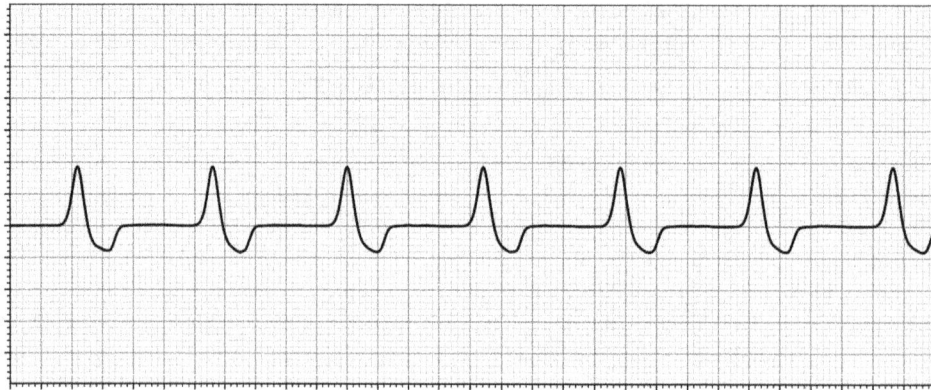

1. Ventricular escape
2. VT
3. Accelerated idioventricular rhythm
4. Junctional tachycardia with bundle branch block

63. A client has end-stage renal disease (ESRD). Which of the following diagnostic findings are consistent with ESRD? *Select all that apply.*

1. Decreased creatinine clearance
2. Metabolic acidosis
3. Respiratory acidosis
4. Anemia
5. Hypophosphatemia
6. Hypercalcemia

64. The nurse has used a needle and syringe to add medication to an intravenous (IV) solution. Which of the following actions should the nurse carry out after injecting the medication into the solution?

1. Invert the IV bag briefly.
2. Begin the infusion with no further action.
3. Roll the IV bag back and forth between the hands a few times.
4. Gently shake the IV bag.

65. A client has had a Port-a-Cath inserted in the upper chest and is receiving chemotherapy, but the client is very tense and complains of much discomfort when the port is accessed. Which of the following is the best solution to the client's discomfort?

1. Administer pain medication prior to the treatment.
2. Apply EMLA cream prior to the treatment.
3. Inject a local anesthetic prior to the treatment.
4. Instruct the client in deep-breathing and relaxation techniques.

66. A 9-year-old boy weighing 22 kg is to receive 15 mg of gabapentin per kg of body weight daily in three divided doses to control seizures. How many mg will he receive in each dose? *Record your answer as a whole number.*

_____ mg

67. A client with deficiency of coagulation factors because of liver disease is to receive 10 mL of fresh frozen plasma per kg of body weight. The client's weight is 183 lb (83 kg). How many mL of FFP should the client receive? *Record your answer as a whole number.*

_____ mL

68. The nurse agrees to represent the hospital at a job fair to distribute alcohol-based hand cleansers and provide information on flu prevention. Which of the following does this participation primarily represent?

1. Professional development
2. Community health education
3. Community service
4. Hospital promotion

69. A 7-month-old infant with community-acquired pneumonia (*H. influenzae*) has received a loading dose of azithromycin oral suspension at a dosage of 10 mg/kg of body weight on day 1 in the emergency department. The infant is now to receive 5 mg/kg/day on days 2–5 up to a maximum of 250 mg/day. The infant's weight is 16.5 lb. How many mg should the infant receive on days 2–5? *Record your answer as a number with one decimal point.*

_____ mg

70. In a normal electrocardiogram (ECG), the QRS complex represents which of the following?

1. Ventricular repolarization
2. AV mode depolarization
3. Atrial depolarization
4. Ventricular depolarization

71. The nurse notes that a client has slid down onto the floor, and he is unable to get up. Which of the following is the best method of lifting him?

1. A belt lift
2. A mechanical lift
3. A two-person chicken lift (lifting under the client's arms)
4. A blanket lift

72. A client has been exploring different types of complementary therapies. Which of the following statements by the client indicate a need for education? *Select all that apply.*

1. "I don't need to worry about taking herbs because they're natural."
2. "Acupuncture may help to relieve back pain."
3. "Homeopathic medicine is better for infections than antibiotics."
4. "Relaxation exercises can help to reduce anxiety."
5. "I should check with the doctor before taking herbal preparations."
6. "I've heard that there is an herbal cure for cancer in Mexico."

73. The nurse is monitoring a woman in labor. During which stage of labor does the nurse expect that the woman will become fully dilated (10 cm)?

1. First stage
2. Second stage
3. Third stage
4. Fourth stage

74. An 8-year-old client lives with his married parents, siblings, grandparents, two aunts, and a cousin. Which of the following family types does this situation comprise?

1. Nuclear family
2. Coparenting
3. Extended family
4. Extended kin network

75. A client with breast cancer who has the _BRCA1_ gene, which is transmitted in an autosomal-dominant manner, asks the nurse if her children are likely to inherit the gene. Which of the following information should the nurse provide?

1. Each child has a 25% chance of inheriting the gene.
2. Each child has a 50% chance of inheriting the gene.
3. All children will inherit the gene.
4. No children will inherit the gene.

76. Which of the following orders utilize correct abbreviations? _Select all that apply_.

1. MS 10.0 mg SC stat
2. DSS Q.D.
3. Levothyroxine 0.112 mg daily
4. Acetaminophen 650 mg at HS
5. TCN 500 mg BID

77. Epinephrine is supplied for a nebulizer inhaler in a dosage of 1:100. What is the percentage strength of the solution? _Record your answer as a whole number._

_____ %

78. A client receiving chemotherapy for breast cancer is to receive metoclopramide HCl at the dosage of 2 mg/kg of body weight 30 minutes before chemotherapy. If the client weighs 55 kg and the medication is provided at 5 mg/mL, how many mL of medication should the client receive? _Record your answer as a whole number._

_____ ml

79. The nurse is assessing an elderly client with severe nausea and vomiting for dehydration. Which of the following signs and symptoms are indicative of dehydration? _Select all that apply_.

1. Urinary specific gravity of 1.006
2. Decrease in hemoglobin and hematocrit
3. Poor skin turgor
4. Dry mucous membranes
5. Decreased thirst
6. Weakness and dizziness

80. The nurse is instructing a client with Addison's disease (adrenocortical insufficiency) about the signs and symptoms of Addisonian crisis. Which of the following should the nurse include? *Select all that apply.*

1. Hypertension
2. Pallor
3. Bradycardia
4. Nausea and abdominal pain
5. Tachycardia
6. Confusion and restlessness

81. A client is to have continuous measuring of his oxygen saturation with a pulse oximeter. However, he has a constant tremor in both of his hands and tends to pick at the covers. Which of the following is the best solution?

1. Apply the oximeter to the little finger because the tremors will not interfere.
2. Apply the oximeter to the little finger, and tape it in place.
3. Advise the physician that pulse oximetry is not possible.
4. Apply an earlobe oximeter.

82. The nurse has recorded a neonate's weight and length in the metric system. The length is recorded as 52.5 cm, but the mother asks how long that is in inches. How many inches are equal to 52.5 cm? *Record your answer as a whole number.*

_____ in

83. The nurse is completing the health history with a client, and he appears obviously uncomfortable when the nurse asks questions about his sexuality. Which of the following is the best method of dealing with the client's discomfort?

1. Acknowledge the client's discomfort in a supportive manner.
2. Make a casual joke, stating that everyone feels discomfort talking about personal issues.
3. Stop asking about sexuality and continue with the next part of the history.
4. Ignore the client's discomfort.

84. The nurse is preparing a client for a mastectomy to treat her breast cancer. Which of the following should the nurse include in the preoperative teaching? *Select all that apply.*

1. Wound care
2. Lymphedema control
3. Deep-breathing and coughing exercises
4. Preoperative restrictions on eating and drinking
5. Instruction regarding the use of patient-controlled analgesia (PCA)

85. When doing nasotracheal suctioning, during which of the following should the catheter be inserted?

1. Inhalation
2. Exhalation
3. Swallowing
4. Coughing

86. Which pain assessment tool is the most appropriate to use with an adolescent?
    1. Face, Legs, Activity, Cry, Consolability (FLACC) scale
    2. Wong–Baker FACES pain rating scale
    3. Children's Hospital of Eastern Ontario Pain Scale (CHEOPS)
    4. One-to-ten scale

87. The nurse is caring for a client with a spinal cord injury at T3, and the client is showing signs and symptoms of autonomic dysreflexia. The client uses intermittent clean catheterization and is due for a scheduled catheterization. In what order should the following interventions be completed?

    I. Loosen any constrictive clothing.
    II. Check the bladder and catheterize the client.
    III. Check for fecal impaction.
    IV. Check the blood pressure (BP) and pulse.
    V. Check the BP and administer a rapid-acting antihypertensive agent if the systolic BP is ≥150 mmHg.

Place the interventions (in Roman numerals) in the correct order from first to last.

    1. ____
    2. ____
    3. ____
    4. ____
    5. ____

88. A client with pancreatic cancer is prescribed fentanyl patches to control pain. Which statement by the client indicates the need for more education?
    1. "The patch will give better pain control if I apply heat over it."
    2. "I should rotate the sites of administration."
    3. "I can dispose of the patch by rolling it up and flushing it down the toilet."
    4. "I should cover the patch with plastic when showering."

89. The unit supervisor assigns a nurse to three clients for primary care, but the nurse discovers that one of the clients is a close neighbor and casual friend. Which of the following is the most appropriate action?
    1. Care for the patient as assigned.
    2. Ask the client if the assignment is acceptable.
    3. Informally ask another nurse to trade clients.
    4. Ask the supervisor to reassign the client.

90. A client involved in a motorcycle accident has a complete spinal cord injury at level C8. Which of the following functional abilities would the nurse expect to observe?
    1. The client requires an electric wheelchair with breath or head controls and assistance with all activities of daily living (ADLs).
    2. The client is able to use a manual wheelchair on level surfaces only, and she can shave, brush her hair, and feed herself with adaptive equipment.
    3. The client is able to use a manual wheelchair on most surfaces, and she is independent in transferring and personal care.
    4. The client requires an electric wheelchair with hand controls, and she is able to feed herself with adaptive equipment.

91. A client with end-stage liver disease is to be discharged from the acute care hospital to his home; however, the client has stated he does not want hospice and that his family will care for him. Which of the following is the most appropriate response?

1. Tell the client that he is placing too large a burden on his family.
2. Advise the client that he is making a mistake.
3. Insist that the client reconsider and accept hospice care.
4. Provide information about the benefits of hospice.

92. A client with fourth-stage cancer of the colon tells the nurse that he has opted to receive no treatment, even though his life may be prolonged with surgery and chemotherapy, because he feels that the emotional and financial costs to himself and to his family are too high. Which of the following responses is most appropriate for the nurse to make?

1. "I hope you will reconsider."
2. "I'm sure your family would rather bear the emotional and financial costs than to lose you."
3. "The palliative care and hospice program can help you with comfort measures, such as pain control."
4. "I think you've made the right decision."

93. A client with a new hearing aid complains of acoustic feedback—whistling—that prevents him from hearing. What should the nurse advise as the initial step to relieve the feedback?

1. Turn down the volume.
2. Remove the hearing aid and reinsert it to ensure it is fit correctly.
3. Decrease the high-frequency amplification.
4. Change the battery.

94. Following the death of a client, the nurse anticipates that rigor mortis will begin in what period of time?

1. 4–6 hours
2. 2–4 hours
3. 1–2 hours
4. 30–60 minutes

95. A client hospitalized for cocaine overdose has removed his intravenous line and is putting on his clothes, stating that he intends to leave the hospital immediately even though he has no discharge order. Which of the following actions is the best response?

1. Tell the client that he is not allowed to leave.
2. Call security to detain the client.
3. Restrain the client.
4. Ask the client to sign the release for leaving against medical advice (AMA).

96. If a client has expressed a desire to quit smoking and asks the nurse for advice, what is the first step that the nurse should suggest?

1. Throw away cigarettes.
2. Ask family members to provide support.
3. Make a quit plan.
4. Sign a contract agreeing to quit.

97. A client has been diagnosed with Parkinson's disease. Which of the following findings would the nurse expect to observe? *Select all that apply.*

1. Resting tremor (unilateral)
2. Flaccidity
3. Hyperkinesia
4. Postural instability
5. Dysphagia
6. Flat affect

98. The nurse is to do chest physiotherapy on an 8-year-old child with cystic fibrosis. Which lobes of the lung are being treated if the child is lying prone with a pillow under the abdomen and lower legs and percussion is administered at the base of the scapulae and immediately inferior to the scapulae?

1. Posterior segments of the right and left upper lobes
2. Anterior segments of the right and left lower lobes
3. Superior segments of the right and left lower lobes
4. Apical segments of the right and left upper lobes

99. What is the nurse's primary responsibility related to continuous quality performance improvement?

1. The nurse should cooperate with measures designed to improve performance.
2. The nurse should be informed about methods of continuous quality performance improvement.
3. The nurse should actively seek methods to improve performance.
4. The nurse should help evaluate outcomes of quality performance improvement measures.

100. A client with chronic lower back pain asks the nurse if she might benefit from some type of complementary therapy. Which of the following complementary therapies should the nurse discuss with the client? *Select all that apply.*

1. Massage
2. Aromatherapy
3. Homeopathy
4. Acupuncture
5. Visualization and relaxation

Answer Key and Explanations for Test #2

Case Study 1

1. 2, 3, 6, and 8: The client's dyspnea with cough, low pulse oximetry reading, and pulse/respirations/blood pressure all require immediate follow-up because they are indicative of respiratory distress, which can quickly escalate to respiratory failure if left without intervention. These factors, in conjunction with the client's history of COPD, support the client's risk for rapid respiratory decline. Although clients with COPD generally have lower oxygen saturation, 86% is low even in this context and must be addressed. A barrel-shaped appearance to the chest is normal in clients with chronic COPD due to the hyperinflation of the lungs secondary to air trapping in the alveoli, and it does not represent an emergent condition. The client's fasting blood glucose was within normal parameters. The client's warm, dry skin is also a normal finding. Although the client's anxiety and productive cough should be addressed and treated, they are not of immediate concern.

2. 2: The client is demonstrating the signs and symptoms of respiratory distress, which could lead to respiratory failure if left untreated. These include dyspnea at rest, decreased oxygen saturation, tachypnea, and wheezing. COPD disrupts the body's ability to properly ventilate due to the air trapping that occurs in the lungs. This can result in a buildup of carbon dioxide (CO_2) because it is not being released. An increase in CO_2 secondary to insufficient ventilation results in respiratory acidosis, which is a complication of COPD exacerbations.

3.

- Administer oxygen, 4 L/min via nasal cannula.
- Chest x-ray.
- Administer albuterol nebulization treatment.
- Collect samples for laboratory tests: sputum culture, complete blood count (CBC), and arterial blood gas (ABG).

The client's oxygen saturation level has decreased, and his overall respiratory status has declined (evidenced by the tripod position and the client only being able to speak one word at a time). The highest priority intervention is to administer oxygen in order to increase his oxygen saturation level and support his respiratory efforts. The nebulization treatment is a priority because it will help open up the client's airway and treat his dyspnea. The sputum culture and CBC will reveal if the client has an infection, and the ABG will demonstrate the severity of the client's respiratory status. The x-ray is not a priority intervention because it will not have an immediate effect on the client's respiratory status and can be performed once the client has been stabilized.

4. 4 and 2: The client's COPD exacerbation has resulted in respiratory acidosis demonstrated by his elevated $PaCO_2$ and decreased pH readings. The kidneys are attempting to compensate for the acidosis by retaining HCO^3 (demonstrated by a slightly elevated HCO^3 level), but they are unable to do so because the pH level remains below normal. This leaves the client with uncompensated respiratory acidosis. The most effective treatment of respiratory acidosis is bilevel positive airway pressure (BiPAP), which assists in opening the alveoli and releasing the trapped air. This would be done prior to invasive mechanical ventilation. Increasing oxygen via nasal cannula would be insufficient, and extracorporeal membrane oxygenation is not indicated unless the patient continues to decline with a pH of less than 7.2.

5.

Potential Nursing Interventions	Indicated	Not Indicated
Anticipate an order for a Foley catheter.	○	●
Assist the client into a supine position.	○	●
Apply a bordered foam dressing to protect the client's skin.	●	○
Educate the client and family on the reasoning for using BiPAP.	●	○
Monitor the patient for abdominal distension.	●	○

There is no indication for a Foley catheter at this time: A bedpan or urinal could be used to avoid introducing infection risks. Moving the client into a supine position will put more pressure on his lungs, and it may worsen his current respiratory status. The client is at risk for skin breakdown related to the pressure caused by the BiPAP mask. Applying a bordered foam dressing to the client's skin will help protect it. It is important to explain the use of BiPAP to the client and family in order to lessen anxiety and ensure understanding of the purpose of the device. The client and family should be informed of the importance of removing excess CO_2 and increasing oxygenation. The client should be monitored for abdominal distension—a potential complication from BiPAP that may cause discomfort.

6.

Assessment Findings	Improved	Unchanged	Worsened
Dyspnea while talking	●	○	○
Respirations, 19	●	○	○
Temperature, 98.5 °F axillary	○	●	○
Pulse oximetry reading, 92%	●	○	○
Heart rate, 121 and irregular	○	○	●
pH, 7.37	●	○	○
PaCO$_2$, 43	●	○	○

During the 1130 assessment, the client was only able to speak one word at a time; however, he is now able to speak in short sentences, which demonstrates improvement of his dyspnea. The client's respiratory rate has decreased from 23 to 19, showing improvement because he is no longer tachypneic. The client remains afebrile; therefore, this component is unchanged. The client's pulse oximetry reading increased from 83% to 92%, which represents an improvement to an acceptable oximetry reading for an individual with COPD. The client's heart rate has increased from 102 to 121, which represents worsening tachycardia. The client's pH and PaCO$_2$ are now within the normal range, which indicates that the client's respiratory acidosis has resolved.

Mometrix

Case Study 2

1. 2, 3, 5, and 6: The client's respiratory rate, work of breathing, and lung sounds all suggest that the client is having trouble moving air. Absent lung sounds on the left could be an indication that the left lung is collapsed. The client's integumentary assessment of cyanotic lips is another indication that he is struggling to perfuse enough oxygen. The client's EKG findings are important, but sinus tachycardia is an expected finding in a client in respiratory distress. His height and weight may also be useful assessment data to assist in diagnosing a potential cause, but this information is not the priority in life-saving treatment and can be considered secondary or tertiary after addressing his breathing difficulties.

2. 4: The client is most likely experiencing a spontaneous pneumothorax. This occurs most commonly without a traumatic cause in young male clients who are tall and thin. The client's sudden-onset chest pain, difficulty breathing, and absent unilateral breath sounds are also indicators of pneumothorax. Although if left untreated, the client could develop tension pneumothorax, his assessment findings do not indicate that at this time. Typical additional signs and symptoms of a tension pneumothorax are tracheal deviation, jugular vein distension, and decreased blood pressure. If tension pneumothorax is suspected, immediate decompression is indicated to prevent shock and cardiac arrest. Although myocardial infarction should be considered given the client's chest pain and shortness of breath (dyspnea), this is less likely given the expected EKG findings and the client's age and medical history. An asthma exacerbation could also be considered to be a cause of the client's dyspnea. However, this would more likely cause wheezing in the lungs (not unilateral absence of breath sounds) and would possibly respond to nebulizer treatment. An anxiety attack could also cause tachycardia, chest pain, and dyspnea in a client. However, this should only be considered if all other likely medical causes are ruled out.

3.

- Obtain a chest x-ray.
- Obtain an arterial blood gas (ABG) reading.
- Administer supplemental oxygen.
- Administer IV morphine.
- Start a second large-bore IV.
- Obtain a repeat EKG.

Of these orders, administering supplemental oxygen is the nurse's top priority. Although the client's pulse oximetry is currently within normal limits, he is clearly in respiratory distress and supplemental oxygen will help him until further intervention is possible. The chest x-ray, ABG, and repeat EKG are necessary to confirm the cause of the client's symptoms. The sooner they are completed, the sooner the correct life-saving interventions can be initiated. Relieving the client's pain with morphine is important, but it is not as high a priority because it is not a life-saving intervention. Similarly, starting a second IV might be necessary to improve access for possible resuscitation, but it is of lower priority because it is not facilitating immediate life-saving measures. The nurse should not spend much time focusing on getting a second IV in when the client is currently struggling to breathe.

4.

Potential Nursing Interventions	Indicated	Not Indicated
Prepare to intubate.	○	●
Prepare the client for the cardiac catheterization lab.	○	●
Prepare for chest tube placement.	●	○
Request an order for further analgesia.	●	○
Prepare for cardioversion.	○	●

Chest tube placement is the indicated treatment for pneumothorax. This procedure can be painful because it involves the physician making an incision into the pleural space and insertion of the chest tube. Thus, additional analgesia is indicated for this relatively stable client. Intubation is not currently indicated because, based on the assessment findings, vitals, and ABG results, the client is maintaining his airway. The cardiac catheterization lab would more likely be indicated if the client was suspected to be having a myocardial infarction, which has been ruled out with EKG. Cardioversion is not indicated for sinus tachycardia. This would be indicated if the client was in supraventricular tachycardia.

5.

Assessment Findings	Improved	Unchanged	Worsened
Pain, 3/10	●	○	○
Respirations, 22	●	○	○
Blood pressure, 90/76	○	○	●
Pulse oximetry, 95%	○	●	○
Integumentary assessment	●	○	○

The client's pain level has decreased, his respiratory rate is closer to normal, and his integumentary assessment is indicating improved oxygenation. The client's blood pressure is now lower than normal parameters. This could be caused by opiate administration, or it could be a sign of shock. The provider should be notified, and further assessments should be conducted. The client's pulse oximetry has increased slightly, but it remains within normal limits.

6. 1 and 3: Seeing a slight change in the water seal level that coordinates with the client's breathing is an expected finding. Also, upon successful placement of the chest tube, the client should have decreased (but regular) work of breathing. Increased work of breathing could be an indication that the chest tube is no longer in place correctly and that the lung has collapsed again due to pneumothorax. Blood should not be found in the chest tube system when it was placed for pneumothorax. The chest tube is meant to drain air from the pleural space. Blood drainage would be an expected finding in a hemothorax. Continuous bubbling in the water seal could be an indication of a leak in the chest tube system. The nurse will need to assess where the leak is and will need to potentially replace the system or notify the physician. The nurse should document the depth that the chest tube is initially placed in the client and ensure that this does not change because it could be an indication of dislodgement. Should there be a significant change in depth, the physician should be notified for possible replacement.

Case Study 3

1. 1, 4, and 5: Any client who has missed a dialysis appointment is at increased risk of fluid overload and electrolyte imbalances. It is important that all dialysis clients understand the danger of missing appointments. The client's serum potassium is critically high and should be the nurse's top concern in this case because it could lead to deadly outcomes. The client's elevated blood pressure (along with the swelling in her limbs) is also concerning, as it shows a sign of possible fluid overload caused by missing her dialysis appointment the day before. The nurse should continue to monitor the patient for further increases in blood pressure because severely high blood pressures can lead to hypertensive emergencies and stroke. Although the client's serum glucose is elevated, this is not a level that is considered critical in most diabetic clients. The client's serum creatinine is also elevated, but this is expected in a renal failure client (especially in those due for dialysis). The client's troponin level is currently within normal limits and is not concerning.

2. 4: Because of the client's missed dialysis appointment and critically high potassium level, the client is currently at highest risk of developing a cardiac arrhythmia such as ventricular tachycardia, ventricular fibrillation, or even asystole. It is critical that this risk is addressed first to prevent cardiac arrest. Although the client is having chest pain and has an abnormal EKG, her troponin is normal, revealing that the peaked T-waves are more likely caused by elevated potassium than a blockage in the heart. Therefore, myocardial infarction is unlikely. Diabetic ketoacidosis is also unlikely given that the client's blood sugar is not critically high for an adult with diabetes and her other assessment findings (normal mentation and breathing) do not suggest this. Additional labs, such as blood gases, would be indicated to further rule out diabetic ketoacidosis. Finally, congestive heart failure may eventually occur in the client that is fluid overloaded, but this is a lower risk because it is generally a chronic condition and treatment is not as emergent for this potential complication.

3.

- Obtain a computed tomography (CT) scan of the abdomen with contrast.
- Administer IV dextrose and insulin.
- Administer IV calcium.
- Administer IV ondansetron.
- Obtain a chest x-ray.

Emergent treatment of the client's elevated potassium is indicated at this time. This is done by administering IV insulin, which can allow the excess serum potassium to pass through the cell membrane. IV dextrose is necessary to prevent the likely hypoglycemia that IV insulin administration can cause. IV calcium is also given in these cases to decrease the risk of cardiac arrhythmia. Although the physician may want a CT scan of the client's abdomen to diagnose a possible cause of her abdominal pain, this diagnosis is not as emergent as preventing potential cardiac arrhythmias from the hyperkalemia. Additionally, the nurse may want to question this order because CT contrast can be nephrotoxic and may cause further damage to the client's already injured kidneys. IV ondansetron may be indicated to help the client feel more comfortable with less nausea, but it is not emergently needed at this time. A chest x-ray may also be indicated to rule out pulmonary edema due to fluid overload. However, the client is not currently presenting with signs of respiratory distress, so this intervention can be delayed.

4.

Potential Nursing Interventions	Indicated	Not Indicated
Request an order for a fluid bolus.	○	●
Request an order for a repeat basic metabolic panel.	●	○
Recheck at the bedside the serum glucose.	●	○
Start a second IV in the left arm.	○	●
Provide continuous cardiac monitoring.	●	○

The client's basic metabolic panel (which includes serum potassium) and serum glucose should be monitored periodically after the administration of IV insulin. This is to ensure that the treatment was effective and to ensure that the client does not become hypoglycemic. Continuous cardiac monitoring is also indicated to monitor for signs that the client's rhythm is worsening or improving. Although the nurse may believe that an IV fluid bolus could help the decrease the client's serum potassium, this is not indicated for a client who is already fluid overloaded. Nurses should always be cautious in administering too much fluid to clients with conditions such as renal failure or congestive heart failure because this can lead to pulmonary edema. Starting a second IV may be a good idea for this client so that more than one medication can be administered at a time in case of emergency. However, it is contraindicated to start an IV in an arm that has a fistula and the nurse should look elsewhere for additional IV access. The nurse should also document the limb restriction in the client's chart and place her on limb restriction precautions, such as placing a "restricted limb" bracelet on the limb, to prevent other healthcare professionals from manipulating that side unknowingly.

5.

Assessment Findings	Improved	Unchanged	Worsened
Glucose, 75	○	○	●
Troponin, 0.01	○	●	○
Potassium, 5.2	●	○	○
Client's neurological assessment	●	○	○
Client's gastrointestinal assessment	●	○	○

Although the client's serum glucose is now considered within normal limits for the average adult, it has dropped significantly since the IV insulin was administered. To prevent further dropping and hypoglycemia, the nurse should encourage glucose intake. If possible, the client should be given food and a sugary beverage. If the physician states that this is contraindicated or it is not safe for the client to take things by mouth, the nurse should advocate for further IV dextrose administration. The client's troponin is slightly higher than the initial reading, but it is still considered normal and is thus considered unchanged. The client's potassium is still elevated and requires intervention, but it is much closer to the normal range and has improved. The client is now no longer too weak to get up; thus, her neurological assessment has improved. Finally, the client is requesting food, which is a likely indication that her nausea and abdominal pain (gastrointestinal assessment) have improved.

6. 1, 2, and 5: While the client's potassium level has improved with the insulin administration, it is still important to monitor for signs of arrhythmias and to continue to check her potassium levels. Insulin is a temporary fix, and potassium levels can rebound if the cause of hyperkalemia is not treated. Therefore, the client should have dialysis soon. An insulin drip is not indicated for this client. In fact, given the drop in her glucose after one dose of IV insulin, an insulin drip would likely be contraindicated. This treatment is meant more for clients with critically high glucose levels. Finally, although IV furosemide may help decrease the client's potassium and fluid overload through her urine, this medication is unlikely to be ordered for a renal client with such a high creatinine level. Furosemide can be nephrotoxic and should be used with caution in this case.

Standalone Questions

1. 3: The appendix is located in the right lower quadrant of the abdomen. In a patient with presumed appendicitis, pain should be expected in this region. The pain often initiates closer to the umbilicus and then moves outward in the right lower quadrant. The pain is often described as sharp and stabbing, worsened by movements such as coughing and sneezing. The patient may also be experiencing nausea and vomiting, fever, abdominal distention, and the inability to pass gas.

2. 2: The nurse should immediately notify the radiation department and make no attempt to touch or move the radiation source. Nurses caring for the client should minimize their time in the room and maximize the distance from the source of radiation (such as standing at the door instead of next to the bed to speak with the client). Although the client should have all necessary care, the nurse must avoid excessive exposure to radiation and may be required to wear appropriate shielding. Nurses who are pregnant should not be involved in care of clients undergoing radiation therapy.

3. 1: Primary graft dysfunction (reperfusion injury) is a major cause of illness and death in lung recipients with symptoms and treatment similar to acute respiratory distress syndrome (ARDS). Indications of primary graft dysfunction include frequent oxygen desaturation, general malaise, increased dyspnea and work associated with the act of breathing, and intolerance to activity. Causes may include increased capillary permeability, interrupted lymphatic drainage, edema, and mismatch in compliance and vascular resistance between the donor and the recipient.

4. 4: If a client with preeclampsia experiences a seizure (indicating eclampsia), the client should be placed in the most protective position for herself and the fetus, the left lateral position. This position decreases the risk that she will aspirate, and it relieves the pressure of the uterus against the vena cava, increasing blood flow to the fetus. The side rails should be raised if the client is in bed, but they should be padded with a blanket or pillows to prevent her from injuring herself.

5. 1: The most common route of entry of microbial agents into the lungs is aspiration. Most aspiration does not result in pneumonia, depending on the microbial load and the patient's condition, because a healthy lung is able to handle small amounts of aspirant. Inhalation is also a common route, either from people who are infected or from contaminated equipment. Vascular spread (bacteremia) is fairly rare but can occur, resulting in pneumonia. In some cases, bacteria and toxins may translocate from the GI system to the lungs per the mesenteric lymph nodes.

6. 4: The best solution is to use an "I" statement to convey the message that the conversation is inappropriate without being accusing: "I don't feel comfortable violating a client's privacy." If an organization is to maintain an ethical environment, then every member of the staff must be willing to address the issue when it arises so others may understand that gossiping about clients is not acceptable behavior.

7. 4: The best solution to an influx of clients during an emergency situation is to carry out early discharge for low-risk, noncritical clients. Often, elective procedures, such as ambulatory surgeries and testing, are canceled and rescheduled. Clients may be sent home with home health care or transferred to other facilities, such as convalescent hospitals. Each facility should have a disaster plan in place that outlines the steps to take in an emergency.

8. 1, 3: Prophylaxis for sickle cell anemia includes penicillin (usually for the first 5 years) to prevent pneumonia and hydroxyurea to promote development of fetal hemoglobin, which helps to prevent sickling of red blood cells. Blood transfusions are not generally given routinely, although a few clients with high risks of stroke, acute chest syndrome, or a ruptured spleen may receive them routinely. Transfusions are more commonly used when anemia worsens or complications such as an enlarged spleen occur. Oxygen is administered when complications such as acute chest syndrome occur.

9. 2, 3, 4, 5: Hard or solid foods that are round pose the greatest risk to children (1–3 years of age) because they can easily asphyxiate if the food becomes lodged in the throat. These foods include peanuts, popcorn, round hard candies, and hot dogs. For the same reason, small children should not have access to coins or other small objects that they might put in their mouths and accidentally swallow. Aspiration of foreign objects is the leading cause of accidental death in infants.

10. 2, 3, 5: Although walking is a healthy exercise, clients with anorexia nervosa often exercise excessively in an effort to lose weight, so jogging in place for extended periods of time at multiple times during the day is a cause for concern. Clients often use laxatives and diuretics to try to induce weight loss, so the nurse should report the client's demand for laxatives. Clients with anorexia frequently experience denial and may become very depressed and withdrawn, and the physician should be notified of this behavior.

11. 1: Because Foley catheters are usually maintained on continuous drainage, the bladder may be essentially empty when it is irrigated, so the small amount of irrigant may pool away from the end of the catheter. Therefore, the best solution if no fluid returns is to turn the client onto the side facing the nurse, being careful to maintain the sterile field. If the irrigant still does not return, then the nurse should gently aspirate using the syringe.

12. 3, 4: Negative pressure wound therapy (NPWT) requires skilled nursing both for removal and application, so these tasks cannot be delegated to UAP nor can wound assessment. However, the nurse should provide instructions to UAP to report any changes in the client's comfort level or any elevation of temperature, as this could indicate infection. Also, the UAP must monitor the tubing to prevent displacement when turning the client.

13. 4: When the suture removal is complete, the nurse should have removed 8 individual pieces of suture. Although the running suture is one long piece of suture material, each stitch in the line must be removed individually. This is because suture material that is on the outside of the skin cannot be pulled through the tissue as it may be contaminated with bacteria.

14: The first action when any type of adverse reaction occurs with a transfusion is to immediately stop the transfusion:

1: (First) II. Stop the transfusion.
2: (Second) I. Notify the physician.
3: (Third) IV. Administer medications (usually antihistamine) as ordered.
4: (Fourth) III. Notify the blood bank.

This type of reaction is classified as a mild to moderate allergic response and may occur during the transfusion and up to an hour after completion of the transfusion and is generally caused by an allergy to a residual plasma protein in the donor's blood.

15. 1: The statement "She purposely hides her belongings from me" suggests that the daughter-in-law believes that the client's behavior is intentional rather than related to confusion. This is a common misconception. Caregivers may blame cognitively impaired clients for their behavior and become angry when the behavior persists. Putting things in the wrong place and forgetting their placement are typical behaviors for clients with Alzheimer's disease. The nurse needs to review behaviors associated with Alzheimer's disease and discuss coping strategies.

16. 1, 2, 3, 4: The Centers for Disease Control (CDC) recommends that adults older than age 65 receive an annual influenza vaccination. The client should receive a pneumococcal vaccination if he has not been previously vaccinated. There are two different types of pneumococcal vaccination: PPSV23 is recommended for those 65 and older, but PCV13 may be recommended according to risk factors as well. Clients should receive a tetanus-diphtheria booster every 10 years. The herpes zoster vaccination is recommended one time for those 60 and older. High-risk clients may be advised to have additional vaccinations.

17. 18: Calculation:

$$\frac{80 \text{ mg}}{15 \text{ mL}} = \frac{96 \text{ mg}}{x \text{ mL}}$$
$$80x = 15 \times 96$$
$$80x = 1{,}440$$
$$8x = 144$$
$$x = \frac{144}{8}$$
$$x = 18$$

The volume needed is 18 mL.

18. 3: Lethargy, change in mental status, and asterixis in a client when receiving TPN are indications of hyperammonemia, so the protein concentration of the formula should be decreased, and the client should be evaluated for hepatic insufficiency. Other complications include insertion trauma, thrombus formation, phlebitis, fluid imbalance, hyperglycemia, hypoglycemia, electrolyte imbalance, azotemia, essential fatty acid deficiency, and hyperlipidemia. Formulas that are commercially prepared contain dextrose and protein, but other trace elements, electrolytes, and vitamins are added as well as fat emulsions on an individual basis.

19. 1, 4, 5, 6: Any radiation treatments to the abdominal area may result in damage to the cells of the small and large intestines, causing diarrhea. The client should be advised to drink ample amounts (8–12 cups) of clear liquid each day and to avoid large meals in favor of five to six small meals daily, which may be better tolerated. Clients may develop rectal irritation, so they should use baby wipes instead of toilet paper or use a squirt bottle with water to cleanse the rectal area. Clients should avoid milk products, fatty foods, gas-producing foods, and fried foods. Imodium is often prescribed to reduce diarrhea.

20. 1: The best response to this client is: "I don't believe she was a match." While the sister is physically matched, she is not emotionally matched. Because people often feel coerced into donating, the United Network for Organ Sharing (UNOS) has provided guidelines that state that potential donors who do not want to donate should receive a nonspecific statement of unsuitability.

21. 4: The most effective method of reducing the spread of nosocomial infections, such as *Clostridioides difficile*, is by practicing a thorough and consistent handwashing routine. The hands may be routinely decontaminated with alcohol-based hand rubs or antimicrobial soap and water. If the hands are visibly dirty or contaminated with body fluids (feces, urine, blood, or sputum), then they should be washed under running water with soap. The hands should be decontaminated before and after direct contact with clients and donning gloves.

22. 3: The most likely reason for these complications is a pneumothorax or bleeding. The nurse should immediately assess the client's lungs to determine if the breath sounds are diminished and notify the physician of the changes in condition. The physician will likely order a chest x-ray and a hemoglobin and hematocrit.

23. 4: The hand is used for palpation, but different parts of the hand are sensitive to different things. The dorsum (back surface) of the hand is most sensitive to variations in skin temperature, such as may occur during an infection or fever. The palm of the hand is used to detect vibrations, such as on the chest wall. The fingertips are very sensitive to shape and texture and are also used to assess pulsations, such as the radial and carotid pulses.

24. 4: The apical pulse is assessed at the fifth left intercostal space at the midclavicular line, which is the point of maximal impulse. The nurse first locates the sternal notch, and from there the second intercostal space. Then, moving fingers lightly down the side of the sternum to the fifth intercostal space and over to the midclavicular line, the nurse should be able to auscultate the S1 and S2 normal heart sounds.

25. 2: Current guidelines advise women ages 40–64 to have Pap smears every two to three years. If Pap smears have been negative for three consecutive years, then many physicians recommend three-year intervals; however, pelvic exams may be done more frequently to assess for other abnormalities or disorders, such as chlamydia or other sexually transmitted diseases. Women who have undergone a total hysterectomy may be advised that they no longer need Pap smears because of removal of the cervix.

26. 4: Any time an object has penetrated the eye, it should be left as undisturbed as possible until the client can be examined by an ophthalmologist because removing the object may cause more damage to the eye. Applying a patch or irrigating the eye may disturb the object as well and should be avoided. The client should be positioned on his back with his head elevated, and he may need medication for pain or relaxation while awaiting the consult. A gauze pad may be placed below the eye if tearing is excessive.

27. 1: The Tensilon (edrophonium chloride) test is used to diagnose myasthenia gravis. Tensilon is an anticholinesterase medication used to increase levels of acetylcholine at the myoneural junctions to relieve symptoms. For the test, the patient is given an injection of Tensilon. If the symptoms are relieved, then the test is positive for myasthenia gravis. If the symptoms remain the same or worsen, then the test is negative. Tensilon is also used to determine if the client is under- or overmedicated with anticholinesterase.

28. 1: If pregnancy is viewed as a natural rather than a medical condition, then pregnant women often seek prenatal care later and less frequently than typical American women. However, the women from other cultures usually follow cultural traditions related to pregnancy, such as restrictions on types of food or activities. They may also seek the advice of older family members or shamans, so lack of prenatal care does not mean that the pregnancy has not been considered or is necessarily at risk.

29. 1: Oral steroids should never be abruptly discontinued and replaced by inhaled steroids because the inhaled steroids alone produce lower plasma levels than the oral preparations. Tapering allows the adrenal glands to recover and function properly. The prednisone dosage should be tapered while the inhaled steroid is introduced to avoid exacerbation of the client's COPD. Clients who have been on oral steroids for extended periods of time may have difficulty with the transition to inhaled steroids and must be monitored carefully.

30. 2, 3, 5: Clients who have previously attempted violent suicide, such as with a gun or knife; who attempted suicide at an isolated site with little chance of rescue; or who have a current history of mental illness and disordered thinking are at a high risk for suicide. Other risk factors include current mental illness and lack of an adequate social support system. Clients with these risk factors should be monitored carefully. Anyone who has previously attempted suicide in any manner has an increased risk of making another attempt.

31. 2: The most likely reason for these symptoms is that the client is experiencing mild pacemaker syndrome. This occurs when the timing of atrial and ventricular contractions is not adequately synchronized. With moderate pacemaker syndrome, the client may experience increased dyspnea, orthopnea, dizziness, and confusion. With severe pacemaker syndrome, the client may develop pulmonary edema and heart failure.

32. 4: Although each person grieves differently, this client's grieving behavior is distorted because she is in a state of prolonged despair that prevents her from working through her grief and finding some resolution. Distorted responses to grief often derive from profound unresolved anger, directed toward oneself, and this can prevent the person from functioning. Clients who had ambivalent feelings toward the deceased may experience prolonged grieving because of guilt and may begin to blame themselves for the person's death.

33. 2: "The company is exempt from the provisions of the ADA because of its size" is the correct response because small businesses employing 15 or fewer employees are not required to comply with the provisions of the ADA even though cancer is considered to be a disability. However, the client should be encouraged to discuss her needs with her employer because some may be willing to make reasonable accommodations. The ADA (1990) is intended to protect persons with disabilities against discrimination. The ADA was amended in 2008.

34. 2: Total patient care is when a nurse is assigned to do all of the care for only one or two clients. Modified primary care is when a nurse is responsible for the same group of clients every day, usually with assistive personnel. Team nursing involves a team leader overseeing a group that comprises unlicensed assistive personnel, licensed vocational/practical nurses, and other registered nurses (RNs) to care for a fairly large group of clients, often ranging from 10 to 20 clients. Functional nursing is when tasks are divided between nurses; for example, one nurse may give medications to all clients, and another nurse might do all the dressing changes.

35. 1: Confused clients with Alzheimer's disease should be placed in a private room to minimize disturbances to other clients. The client should be near the nursing station and within the nurses' line of sight so a close watch can be kept over the client. Restraints should be avoided if at all possible because they often cause clients to become more agitated. Clients who are confused and trying to climb out of bed may require a sitter during hospitalization.

36. 3: The best position for a client with impaired swallowing is upright with the head midline and the chin down (flexed about 75% of the way toward the chest) because this position provides better protection of the airway and decreases the risk of choking and aspirating. The patient may be positioned with the arms on the overbed table with positioning aids used, if necessary, to maintain body alignment. The client should continue to remain in the upright position for at least 30 minutes after the feeding is completed.

37. 2: If monitoring a client's control of diabetes, the most reliable source of information is the client's HbA1c, which indicates the average level of glucose over a 3-month period. The serum glucose level can change from day to day depending on carbohydrate intake and various other factors, so it is less reliable. While the client's diet and exercise log provide valuable information, clients are not always accurate or honest with reports.

38. 2: According to federal law, if a client dies in a hospital setting, the staff must ask the family decision maker about organ donation. In some cases, the client will have indicated a preference on an advance directive. However, in practice, if family members object, the harvesting of organs is usually not carried out. It is important that the staff member approaching the family be trained and sensitive to the family members' feelings and concerns. Information about organ donation is often provided to the client and family on admission.

39. 1, 2, 4, 5: Clients need adaptive equipment to allow them to be independent in their own care and to prevent injury to the hip during the healing process. Equipment that is considered to be necessary on discharge includes a walker, an elevated toilet seat, a reacher/grabber to pick things up, and a sock aid to assist the client with getting dressed. Most clients should not need a wheelchair after discharge unless they have comorbidities. Although some clients may be ready to use a cane on discharge, most are still dependent on walkers, which provide better stability.

40. 1, 2, 3, 5: Typical indications that death will occur within a few days include lethargy, disorientation, and increasing dysphagia. Clients are usually unable to take foods or swallow medications. The client appears very weak, gaunt, and pale and is able to take only sips of fluid. Clients usually have decreased urinary output and may be incontinent of concentrated urine. The cardiac rate and respiratory rate both increase, but the strength of cardiac contractions weakens, and the pulse may become irregular.

41. 2: Timed voiding involves toileting on a regularly scheduled basis, usually every two hours during waking hours and one or two times during the night. This is especially useful for those with cognitive impairment. Bladder training is when toileting is scheduled with progressive voiding intervals, but the client must be cognitively aware. Patterned urge response toileting is a form of habit training that uses an electronic monitoring device. Prompted voiding involves prompting regularly-scheduled toilet breaks for those able to use the toilet independently, such as clients with mild dementia.

42. 1: A common response to severe trauma, such as rape, is denial. Clients may at one extreme deny an event has even happened, but more often they exhibit denial by closing down their emotions and remaining calm, insisting that they are "fine" and need no intervention or help. They may try to appear and function as though the event has not happened at all so they can "get on with their life." This is rarely a good solution because they may not adequately deal with the trauma emotionally, resulting in ongoing psychological problems, such as depression, suicidal ideation, flashbacks, and fear.

43. 1, 3, 4, 5: Most infant abductors are female, approximately age 30, and overweight. They rarely have a criminal record and may appear quite normal, although they may be emotionally immature and behave impulsively. Abductors often visit the site of abduction in advance. They may ask many questions about procedures and nursery policies or try to become friendly with staff and parents to gain information and trust. Abductors often seek to replace a child they have lost or to compensate for their inability to have children.

44. 1, 4: The expected outcomes should relate specifically to the nursing diagnosis (rather than the clinical diagnosis) and interventions:

- Nursing diagnosis: Chronic low self-esteem.
- Intervention 1: Self-esteem enhancement—Help the client identify and review negative perceptions of self. Encourage him to take an active role in his treatment planning.
- Intervention 2: Self-awareness enhancement—Help the client identify personal positive beliefs and characteristics as well as self-limiting behaviors.
- Expected outcomes: The client is able to use positive self-talk to interrupt negative thinking. He is able to use positive coping behaviors to improve his functioning.

45. 1: The client should be advised to avoid sunbathing because tetracycline causes photosensitivity, which can occur immediately upon exposure or sometime after exposure to sunlight. Tetracycline should be taken with a full glass of water 1 hour before or 2 hours after meals. Clients should be cautioned that milk, other dairy products, and iron products reduce the absorption of tetracycline, so they should not be consumed within 2 hours of the drug dosing. Tetracycline should not be given to children younger than 8 years of age.

46. 4: *N*-acetylcysteine is the antidote for an acetaminophen overdose. Acetaminophen toxicity occurs with a single dose greater than 140 mg/kg of body weight or with greater than 7.5 g in 24 hours. The antidote is given for serum levels greater than 150. It is most effective if given with 8 hours of ingestion. *N*-acetylcysteine is given at the rate of 140 mg/kg initially and repeated with 70 mg/kg every 4 hours for 17 additional doses, either by mouth or intravenously.

47. 3: The nurse should instruct the client to open her mouth and hold the inhaler one to two inches in front of her mouth (about two finger widths). The client should exhale and then inhale deeply for 5 seconds while pressing down on the inhaler to release a dose of medication. After inhaling the medication, the client should hold her breath for about 10 seconds and then exhale slowly through pursed lips. Children and those who have difficulty managing the procedure should use spacers.

48. 3: Edema is a common problem related to burns, so the nurse must check peripheral pulses frequently (at least every two hours) and keep the extremities elevated on two pillows. If the pulses become diminished, the first step is to loosen the dressings and recheck the pulses to determine if the dressings are restricting blood flow. Burns are often treated with topical agents and several layers of dressings, which should be applied on the lower extremities distally to proximally.

49. 3: Cholecystitis may result in severe episodes of pain in the right upper quadrant of the abdomen, often lasting two to six hours, and sometimes radiating to the back. Clients may also experience indigestion, nausea and vomiting, and clay-colored stools if the bile duct is blocked. In severe cases, jaundice may be evident. Cholecystitis may result from calculi or pancreatitis and is most common in overweight females ages 20–40, but it also may occur in women who are pregnant.

50. 1, 3, 4: The nurse cannot delegate assessments regarding the initial need for restraints, the ongoing need for restraints, or the type of restraint needed. However, unlicensed assistive personnel may apply restraints (if they have been trained to do so), position clients while they are in restraints, check restraints for correct placement, and provide supportive care, such as toileting and providing fluids and skin care. These actions should be performed under the guidance of the nurse, who should provide clear instructions regarding how long the restraints are to be in place, how frequently the client should be turned, and any other care that should be provided.

51. 4: While a nasogastric tube for decompression is usually placed with the client's head elevated, when gastric lavage is done to remove drugs or poisons, the client is placed in the left lateral position with the head lowered 15 degrees. This position causes the substances in the stomach to pool and reduces movement of the substances into the duodenum. A large bore tube (36–40 Fr) is usually used for gastric lavage and may be placed nasally or orally.

52. 1: The response that demonstrates therapeutic communication is "Your pain is not well controlled" because it is restating the implied message that the client is communicating. The nurse should avoid making "should" statements or questioning the client's actions, but she should attempt to explore the issue to determine what intervention is needed. "You poor thing" is not helpful in solving the problem and suggests that the client is a victim rather than an active collaborator in his own care.

53. 4: With peritoneal dialysis, a typical exchange cycle takes 30–45 minutes and includes three phases: infusion of 2–3 liters of dialysate (5–10 minutes), dwell time (about 10 minutes), and drainage (10–30 minutes). The number of cycles each day is determined on an individual basis. The drainage fluid should be straw-colored or clear. Cloudy drainage may indicate an infection. Blood-tinged drainage may occur shortly after insertion of the abdominal catheter and during menses.

54. 4: The prone position may cause blood to pool in the extremities, and pressure on the abdomen may result in a decrease in blood pressure (BP), preload, and cardiac output. Respiratory effort increases, and lung compliance decreases. The head positioned sharply to one side may interfere with cerebral circulation. If the head is turned laterally, the dependent eye must be observed carefully for external compression. Bilateral bolsters or other supports should be used to support the thorax (clavicle to iliac crest) to relieve abdominal compression, which may impede respirations and venous return.

55. 1, 3, 4: Post-mortem care includes positioning the limbs in proper alignment, placing dentures in the mouth, and cleansing the body gently (because the tissue is friable after death). The eyelids should be closed, but taping or applying weights is not necessary (tape may damage tissue). A roll may be placed under the jaw to hold the mouth closed. The body is usually left unclothed. These interventions should be carried out shortly after death because rigor mortis begins within 2–4 hours.

56. 1: These signs and symptoms indicate hypokalemia. Potassium influences the activity of both skeletal and cardiac muscles. Normal values range from 3.5–5.5 mEq/L. Hypokalemia occurs with levels of less than 3.4 mEq/L and critical values of less than 2.5 mEq/L.

57. 1, 3, 4: The following tests must be performed to diagnose brain death prior to organ donation:

- 2 EEGs are taken 12–24 hours apart to assess electrical activity.
- Brainstem reflexes are tested. These include pupillary response to light, corneal reflex, vestibular ocular reflex, gag reflex, and motor response to pain.
- Apnea tests are usually performed after a second testing of brainstem reflexes, but it only needs to be done once if the results are conclusive.

If injuries are so severe that they prevent some testing, then other confirmatory testing, such as transcranial Doppler ultrasonography, may be done.

58. 4: COPD clients are unable to adequately use accessory muscles of respiration, so leaning forward at 30–40° improves the upward movement of the diaphragm. This allows more air to be expelled with each exhalation and helps to reduce breathlessness. The patient may be positioned with the arms resting on an overbed table if in bed or on the thighs or a small table if sitting in a chair. Many COPD clients sleep sitting up because of increased shortness of breath when they try to recline.

59. 4: The correct dosage in grams is 3 g piperacillin/0.375 g tazobactam. Calculation:

$$(30 \text{ kg}) \times \left(100 \ \frac{\text{mg piperacillin}}{\text{kg}}\right) = 3,000 \text{ mg piperacillin}$$

$$(30 \text{ kg}) \times \left(12.5 \ \frac{\text{mg tazobactam}}{\text{kg}}\right) = 375 \text{ mg tazobactam}$$

To convert milligrams to grams:

$$(3,000 \text{ mg piperacillin}) \times \left(\frac{1 \text{ g}}{1,000 \text{ mg}}\right) = 3 \text{ g piperacillin}$$

$$(375 \text{ mg tazobactam}) \times \left(\frac{1 \text{ g}}{1,000 \text{ mg}}\right) = 0.375 \text{ g tazobactam}$$

60. 1, 2: HIPAA privacy and security rules protect personal health information about a client, so it is a HIPAA violation to share information about the client with family and friends other than parents of a minor child or a spouse without specific permission to do so. It is a security violation to allow unauthorized access to the EHR, and this includes not only sharing passwords but also allowing others to "shoulder surf" in order to gain information.

61. 3: The nurse should telephone the physician to question the dosage and should be prepared to tell the physician the client's weight in kg and the recommended dosage. In some cases, the physician may have a valid reason for exceeding the usual dosage, but the staff should be aware of the reasons. It is the nurse's responsibility to ensure that the five rights of medication administration are adhered to: right client, right drug, right dose, right route, and right time.

62. 3: Accelerated idioventricular rhythm (AIVR) is characterized by:

- Heart rate between 50 and 100 bpm
- Regular or only slightly irregular rhythm
- Wide QRS complex (≥0.12 s)

AIVR can be mistaken for ventricular tachycardia (VT), which is typically faster than 120 bpm. VT is life-threatening, whereas AIVR is typically benign and ends without intervention. AIVR is common after reperfusion therapy and occurs in almost a third of patients. Other triggers for AIVR include potassium imbalance, drug toxicity (e.g., digoxin, flecainide, propafenone), cardiomyopathy, and cardiac arrest with successful resuscitation.

63. 1, 2, 4: Findings consistent with end-stage renal disease (ESRD) include the following:

- Creatinine clearance decreases as glomerular filtration rate decreases, while serum creatinine and blood urea nitrogen (BUN) levels increase.
- Metabolic acidosis results from a decreased ability of the kidneys to excrete ammonia and reabsorb sodium bicarbonate.
- Anemia results from inadequate production of erythropoietin by the kidneys.
- Fluid retention related to hypernatremia increases the risk of heart failure and edema.
- Both hyperphosphatemia and hypocalcemia result from the kidneys not adequately filtering out phosphorus, because phosphorus and calcium concentrations have a reciprocal relationship.

64. 4: After medication is injected into the port of an intravenous bag, it will tend to pool in the lower part of the bag, so the nurse should gently shake the bag to distribute the medication more evenly throughout the solution. The infusion bag must be labeled according to facility policy, usually with the patient's name, room number, name of the medication, date and time the medication is mixed, date and time the infusion is started, and the initials of the nurse administering the infusion.

65. 2: Although the client may benefit from pain medication prior to treatment because of increased pain associated with administration of chemotherapy and may be less tense if instructed in deep-breathing and relaxation exercises, these are not good solutions for the local discomfort associated with port access. The best solution is to apply EMLA (lidocaine/prilocaine) cream to the port area about 20–45 minutes prior to treatment. If receiving chemotherapy as an outpatient, the client can apply the cream and cover the area with plastic wrap before leaving home.

66. 110: Calculation:

$$(22 \text{ kg}) \times \left(\frac{15 \text{ mg gabapentin}}{\text{kg}}\right) = 330 \text{ mg gabapentin}$$

This is the total dosage, but it is to be given in 3 divided doses:

$$330/3 = 110 \text{ mg}$$

67. 830: If a client with deficiency of coagulation factors because of liver disease is to receive 10 mL of fresh frozen plasma per kg of body weight and the client's weight is 183 lb (83 kg), the patient should receive 830 mL of FFP (83 × 10). FFP is usually supplied in 200 mL units, and the required dose is rounded to the nearest unit, so the patient would receive 4 units of FFP. FFP must be ABO/Rh compatible and must be administered within 24 hours of thawing.

68. 2: The nurse is participating in community health education by providing alcohol-based cleansers and educating the public about methods to prevent the flu. Community health education may be formal, with classes scheduled on a number of different health topics, or informal, such as answering questions about health matters and setting an example for others in the community. The nurse often serves as a resource person for others with questions about health matters.

69. 37.5: The first step is to convert the child's weight from pounds to kilograms, and then multiply the weight by the dosage in mg per kg.

$$16.5 \text{ lb} \times \frac{1 \text{ kg}}{2.2 \text{ lb}} = 7.5 \text{ kg}$$

$$(5 \text{ mg/kg}) \times (7.5 \text{ kg}) = 37.5 \text{ mg}$$

70. 4: In the normal electrocardiogram (ECG) complex, the QRS complex represents ventricular depolarization:

- P wave: Start of electrical impulse in the sinus node and spreading through the atria, muscle depolarization
- QRS complex: Ventricular muscle depolarization and atrial repolarization. The width of the complex represents intraventricular conduction time.
- T wave: Ventricular muscle repolarization (resting state) as cells regain negative charge
- U wave: Repolarization of the Purkinje fibers

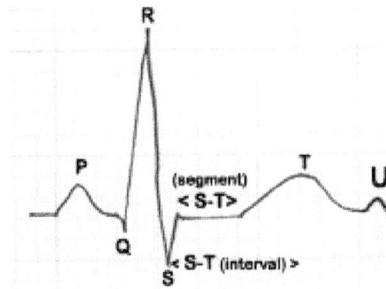

71. 2: The nurse should assist the client into a position of comfort on the floor and use a mechanical lift to raise the client. There is no other lift that will raise the client and not pose a risk of injury to the nurse or those assisting. If the client is fairly mobile and strong, he may be assisted into a four-point position on his knees, and a chair is placed next to him so he can raise himself with minimal assistance.

72. 1, 3, 6: If a client has been exploring different types of complementary therapies and states, "I don't need to worry about taking herbs because they're natural," the client needs to be aware that many prescription medications are derived from herbs, and herbs may interact with medications and increase or decrease their actions. Additionally, "Homeopathic medicine is better for infections than antibiotics," is not supported by any research and may pose a risk to the client if an infection goes untreated. "I've heard that there is an herbal cure for cancer in Mexico" suggests the client is relying on unsubstantiated claims.

73. 1: There are four stages of labor:

Stage 1: The period between the onset of labor and full dilation (10 cm). Comprises two phases: latent (cervical effacement and beginning dilation) and active (continued dilation from 4 to 10 cm).
Stage 2: The period from full dilation through the delivery of the infant.
Stage 3: The period after delivery of the infant through delivery of the placenta.
Stage 4: The postpartum period lasting two hours after delivery.

74. 3: Extended families are multigenerational families or shared households with parents, friends, or other family members, such as aunts and uncles. Nuclear families are considered by many to be the traditional family model, consisting of a mother, a father, and children. Coparenting is when custody is shared between two families, such as with a divorce custody agreement. Extended kin networks are when two nuclear families live together or near each other and share goods and services, such as childcare.

75. 2: When a mother has an autosomal-dominant gene, each child has a 50% chance of inheriting the gene. However, because inheritance is a random process, this does not mean that 50% will actually inherit the gene. In fact, all children or no children may inherit the gene. Humans should have 23 pairs of chromosomes. Pairs 1–22 are autosomal, and pair 23 is sex with XX for female and XY for male.

In the Punnett square below, N represent the normal gene and D represents the dominant mutated gene.

	N	**D**
N	NN	ND (mutation)
N	NN	ND (mutation)

76. 3, 4: The orders that correctly use abbreviations are "Levothyroxine 0.112 mg daily" because the decimal has a leading zero and "acetaminophen 650 mg at HS" because "at" is spelled out rather than using "@," which may be misread as the number 2. The order "MS 10.0 mg SC stat" improperly abbreviates morphine sulfate and has a trailing zero, which can result in the order being misread as "100 mg." "DSS Q.D." uses "Q.D." instead of "daily" or "each day." Abbreviations, such as "TCN" for tetracycline, should be avoided.

77. 1: Epinephrine 1:100 means that there is 1 part medication to 100 parts diluent. This ratio is equivalent to the fraction $\frac{1}{100}$ which is equivalent to 1%.

78. 22: Calculation:

$$(55 \text{ kg}) \times (2 \text{ mg/kg}) = 110 \text{ mg}$$

The medication is provided with 5 mg per mL:

$$\frac{110 \text{ mg}}{5 \text{ mg/mL}} = 22 \text{ mL}$$

79. 3, 4, 6: Dehydration results in the following signs and symptoms:

- Increased urinary specific gravity (>1.028)
- Increased blood urea nitrogen (BUN) and BUN-creatinine ratio
- Increased hemoglobin and hematocrit
- Poor skin turgor
- Dry mucous membranes
- Weakness and dizziness
- Tachycardia
- Fever

Elderly clients are especially susceptible to dehydration, so their fluid intake should be monitored carefully. Rehydration and replacement of lost electrolytes are critical. Clients may be provided oral rehydration fluids or intravenous (IV) fluids, depending on their condition and ability to tolerate oral fluids.

80. 2, 4, 5, 6: Addisonian crisis is an acute episode of adrenal insufficiency that is life threatening and precipitated by a stressor, such as gastrointestinal infection, fever, or surgery. Addisonian crisis may be misdiagnosed as an acute abdomen because clients may present with nausea and severe abdominal pain. Shock, with hypotension and pallor, is common, and clients may exhibit tachycardia, confusion, and restlessness. Because temperature regulation is impaired, clients may exhibit hypothermia or hyperthermia. Suspected Addisonian crisis must be treated immediately because clients may die while awaiting test results.

81. 4: The nurse should apply an earlobe oximeter. A digit pulse oximeter should be avoided if the client has tremors or if he is likely to move his hand frequently. The skin should be clean and dry when the oximeter is applied. If using a digit oximeter, a client should not have artificial nails or wear colored nail polish because these may interfere with readings. If a client is severely obese, the clip on the oximeter may not stay in place, so a disposable (single-use) sensor pad may be necessary.

82. 21: Calculation:

$$(52.5 \text{ cm}) \times \frac{1 \text{ in}}{2.5 \text{ cm}} = 21 \text{ in}$$

83. 1: The best solution to dealing with a client's discomfort is to acknowledge the discomfort in a supportive manner: "I can see that these questions are making you uncomfortable because it's difficult for most people to talk about personal issues." Joking about the client's discomfort or ignoring it altogether shows a lack of respect for the client's feelings, and stopping the questions is not a good solution because the information may be important for providing a full understanding of the client and his health issues.

84. 3, 4, 5: Clients should not be overwhelmed with preoperative instructions, so wound care and lymphedema control should be discussed postoperatively. Because lung ventilation is very important after surgery, the client should practice deep-breathing and coughing exercises preoperatively and should know what food and fluid restrictions (such as no fluids for six hours before surgery) must be complied with. Because clients usually return from surgery with patient-controlled analgesia (PCA) in place, instructions about its use should occur preoperatively when the client is more alert and not yet in pain.

85. 1: When doing nasotracheal suctioning, the catheter should be inserted only during inhalation because this is when the epiglottis is open. However, suction should not be applied during insertion. During suctioning, a normal reaction is for the client to cough, but if the client begins to gag or becomes nauseated, the catheter may be in the esophagus. Tracheal suctioning should be completed before pharyngeal because the pharynx contains more bacteria than the trachea.

86. 4: Unless the adolescent has a cognitive or other physical impairment that interferes with his ability to comprehend, the most appropriate pain assessment tool is the 1-to-10 scale, which is commonly used with adults. The Face, Legs, Activity, Cry, Consolability (FLACC) scale is appropriate for children from 2 months to 7 years of age. The Wong–Baker FACES tool can be used from ages three on up through adulthood, but it is most appropriate for children before adolescence because of its cartoonish nature.

87. Correct order:

1: (First) IV. Check the blood pressure (BP) and pulse.
2: (Second) I. Loosen any constrictive clothing.
3: (Third) II. Check the bladder and catheterize the client.
4: (Fourth) V. Check the BP and administer a rapid-acting antihypertensive agent if the systolic BP is ≥150 mmHg.
5: (Fifth) III. Check for fecal impaction.

Treatment should always begin by checking vital signs (VS), then loosening clothes, and then progressing to the assessment of the bladder. If there is no indwelling catheter, the client should be catheterized. If a catheter is in place, it must be checked for patency and irrigated if necessary. The BP should be checked again, and an antihypertensive agent should be administered if the BP remains elevated before checking for fecal impaction.

88. 1: Clients must avoid placing direct sources of heat, such as a heating pad, over a fentanyl patch because this action increases the rate of absorption and may cause the client to have an overdose. Clients are allowed to bathe or shower while wearing the patch, but this may cause the patch to loosen. To prevent this, clients may cover the patch with plastic wrap taped in place. A patch should be disposed of by rolling it and flushing it down the toilet because some medication will remain in the patch.

89. 4: In this situation, the nurse should immediately inform the supervisor and ask that the client be reassigned. Since the nurse and client have a preexisting social relationship, the client may be uncomfortable with the nurse knowing personal information or providing care but may not be comfortable stating so outright.

90. 2: A client with a complete spinal cord injury at level C8 is a quadriplegic and should be able to use a manual wheelchair independently on most surfaces but may require adaptive devices for activities of daily living (ADLs). The client should have full extension and flexion of her elbows and wrists and some movement in the fingers and thumbs. She should be able to transfer independently and drive a car with hand controls. The client may need some assistance with ADLs, such as lower body dressing.

91. 4: Clients may turn down offers of hospice care because they have no clear idea of the benefits and may mistakenly believe that hospice is just there to provide support during death. The nurse should explain the benefits, such as the provision of equipment, supplies, pain medication, and pain control, as well as services by other supportive members of the hospice team, such as home health aides and social workers. The client should be advised that he can contact hospice at any time if he changes his mind.

92. 3: The most appropriate response to a client who has chosen to receive no treatment is the one that supports the client's choice and provides useful information: "The palliative care and hospice program can help you with comfort measures, such as pain control." The nurse should avoid trying to pressure the client into accepting treatment, and holding out the possibility of a cure for someone with fourth-stage cancer is essentially meaningless. For some clients, having no treatment is the best choice.

93. 2: A frequent cause of acoustic feedback with a hearing aid is incorrect fit, so removing the hearing aid and reinserting it, making sure that it is seated properly in the ear canal, may alleviate the problem. If the acoustic feedback persists, then the client may have earwax or the hearing aid may need to be refitted because the fit may be too loose. In some cases, adjusting the high-frequency amplification may reduce acoustic feedback, but it may also decrease the ability to hear speech, so this is usually not a good solution.

94. 2: Following the death of a client, rigor mortis usually begins within two to four hours because adenosine triphosphate (ATP), which is necessary to relax muscles, is no longer synthesized, so muscles contract. It's important to position the client before rigor mortis begins. This includes closing the eyes, placing dentures in the mouth, closing the jaw (using a rolled towel to keep the mouth closed), positioning the hands, and positioning the body in correct alignment.

95. 4: Unless treatment is court ordered, clients cannot be prevented from leaving the hospital. Telling the client that he cannot leave, calling security, or restraining the client would be to violate his rights to self-determination and could be construed as unlawful imprisonment. The nurse should ask the client to sign the release for leaving against medical advice (AMA) and should follow hospital protocol for such situations. The nurse should ask the client to speak with the physician before leaving.

96. 3: The first step that the nurse should suggest to the client is for them to make a quit plan. The client should determine a quit date, preferably within 2 weeks. During that time, the client should inform family and friends, make a list of possible adverse effects (cravings, withdrawal), and plan a response. The client should review smoking habits (when, where, and how) and make a plan to avoid those situations. On the quit date, the client should throw away all tobacco products.

97. 1, 4, 5, 6: Parkinson's disease is related to deficiency of the neurotransmitter dopamine. Signs and symptoms include resting tremor (usually unilateral initially of the upper extremity, but it may affect the foot or face), rigidity, bradykinesia, postural instability, dysphagia, and flat affect. Clients with Parkinson's disease often walk leaning forward and with a short, shuffling gait with a reduced arm swing. Speech is often slow and slightly slurred with a monotonous tone. Many clients exhibit micrographia (small, illegible writing).

98. 3: In this position, the superior segments of the right and left lower lobes are being treated. Chest physiotherapy (CPT) should not be administered on bare skin. Percussion may be done with a CPT cup for very small children and with cupped hands for older children and adults. Vibration is done after the client takes a deep breath and while he exhales.

99. 3: Although cooperating, being informed, and evaluating outcomes are all important in continuous quality performance improvement, the nurse's primary responsibility is to actively seek methods to improve performance. The nurse must remain current in the profession; evaluate evidence and seek out best practices; observe methods and outcomes; and look for opportunities to make changes, big and small, that may improve the quality of client care and/or improve the cost-effectiveness of care and return on investment.

100. 1, 4, 5: Research has shown that acupuncture and massage may help to reduce chronic lower back pain. Acupuncture is a part of traditional Chinese medicine in which tiny needles are inserted into acupoints and left in place for 30–60 minutes to balance the vital energy. Massage helps to relax the muscles and relieve discomfort. Visualization and relaxation can benefit almost all clients because they can help to reduce anxiety and relax tense muscles. There is no evidence that either aromatherapy or homeopathy is effective in reducing chronic lower back pain.

Practice Test #3

Case Study 1

A 35-year-old male arrives at the emergency department via ambulance.

<u>NURSES' NOTES</u>

1400: A 35-year-old male client is brought into the emergency department via ambulance. The client appears to be grimacing and groaning, and he is clutching his left forearm. Emergency medical services has placed the client's arm in a makeshift splint and has started an IV in the client's right forearm. The client appears to be alert and oriented ×4 and expresses that his pain was initially rated 10/10 until emergency medical services administered 100 mcg of IV fentanyl 15 minutes prior to his arrival at the hospital. The client states that his pain is now 7/10. The client reports that he was riding on a skateboard when he fell to his left side, catching himself with his hands. The client was not wearing a helmet or protective gear. He denies striking his head or losing consciousness, stating that his skateboard hit a pebble on the road. There are abrasions on both of his palms and a laceration on his left wrist. The left wrist appears swollen, with a possible deformity, and the client struggles to move the fingers on his left hand due to the pain. The client denies any medical history or taking any medications. The client is changed into a gown, and his vital signs are obtained.

<u>VITAL SIGNS</u>

	1400
Temp	98.5 °F temporal
HR	110
BP	155/65
RR	22
Pulse oximetry	96% on room air

<u>PHYSICAL ASSESSMENT</u>

Body System	**1400**
Neurological	The client is alert and oriented ×4. Sensation to the injured limb is intact, and the client denies any numbness or tingling. There are no signs of injury to the client's head or neck, and he denies any headache.
Pulmonary	The client is breathing quickly, but his airway is intact. Breath sounds are clear and regular.
Cardiovascular	Heart rate is tachycardic. Heartbeat is strong and regular. Left radial pulse is strong and regular. Capillary refill is <3 seconds.
Integumentary	Abrasions are noted to both palms. There is a laceration to the left wrist, but the bleeding is under control.
Musculoskeletal	The client reports pain to his left wrist and forearm. He has decreased range of motion to his left hand due to pain. Swelling is noted to the left upper extremity. A deformity is noted to the left wrist.

1. From the following list, select the assessment findings that require <u>immediate</u> follow-up. (Select all that apply)

1. Blood pressure, 155/65
2. Heart rate, 110
3. Integumentary assessment
4. Pulmonary assessment
5. Musculoskeletal assessment
6. Mechanism of injury

2. Based on the nurse's assessment findings, the client is <u>most likely</u> experiencing _____.

1. compartment syndrome
2. osteomyelitis
3. an open fracture
4. a dislocation

3. The nurse receives the following orders. Highlight all orders from the following list that the nurse should consider a <u>priority</u>.

- Administer IV cefazolin.
- Obtain urine toxicology results.
- Administer the tetanus, diphtheria, and pertussis (Tdap) vaccine.
- Obtain blood work.
- Obtain an x-ray of the affected limb.
- Educate the client on skateboard safety.

NURSES' NOTES

1420: An x-ray of the client's wrist reveals a displaced fracture to the ulna. The client's wounds are irrigated, and the physician determines that the laceration does not need suturing or closure. The physician orders procedural sedation with Propofol for the reduction and splinting of the bone. The physician discusses the plan with the client and obtains consent to proceed.

4. For the following list of potential nursing interventions, specify whether each is indicated or not indicated.

Potential Nursing Interventions	Indicated	Not Indicated
Place the client on cardiac and capnography monitoring.	O	O
Prepare for intubation.	O	O
Anticipate the administration of an IV fluid bolus.	O	O
Set up bedside suction and bag valve mask.	O	O
Start a second IV on the left forearm.	O	O

NURSES' NOTES

1500: The healthcare team is ready for the procedural sedation and reduction. The nurse has pulled the Propofol from the medication storage unit, the physician is at the bedside with an emergency medical technician ready with splinting supplies, and the respiratory therapist is at the head of the bed. The client is on cardiac and capnography monitoring, and resuscitation supplies

103

are within reach. A procedural time-out is performed, the physician administers the first dose of Propofol, and the client is silent as the physician pulls on the left limb to reduce the fractured ulna. Five minutes after the Propofol is administered, the team notices that the client's vital signs have changed. The 1500 and 1505 vital sign measurements are as follows:

	1500	1505
Temp	98.9 °F temporal	98.6 °F temporal
HR	96	90
BP	145/64	92/40
RR	20	16
Pulse oximetry	95% on room air	87% on room air

5. The nurse anticipates that the physician will instruct the sedation team to _____, _____, and _____. (Select three answers)

1. administer IV naloxone
2. administer supplemental oxygen
3. perform the jaw thrust maneuver
4. administer epinephrine intramuscularly
5. administer an IV fluid bolus
6. start cardiopulmonary resuscitation (CPR)

Nurses' Notes

1510: The interventions were successful, and the client's blood pressure and pulse oximetry readings improved and are now stable. The reduction and splinting are completed. The client's left arm is placed in an ulnar gutter splint. A repeat x-ray is performed, which reveals that the fracture is no longer displaced.

6. After an observation period, the client is now fully awake and has orders for discharge. Of the following statements, which indicate that the client demonstrates an understanding of discharge instructions? (Select all that apply)

1. "If my fingers become painful or numb, I will tighten the elastic bandage of my splint."
2. "I will need to follow up with an orthopedic specialist in the next few days."
3. "I will return to the emergency department if my pain is severe and unrelieved by analgesics."
4. "Fever and purulent drainage are expected for an injury like mine."
5. "I need to wear my sling for the first 24 hours, even when I sleep."
6. "If I take acetaminophen for pain, I should be careful not to exceed 4,000 mg in 1 day."

Case Study 2

The nurse is caring for an 18-year-old male client in the emergency department.

NURSES' NOTES (EMERGENCY DEPARTMENT)

Day 1, 1430: The client arrived at the emergency department today reporting pain in his right arm. He was seen in the hospital yesterday due to injuries sustained in a motor vehicle accident, including a broken nose, a laceration to his chin requiring six stitches, and a fracture to the right ulna requiring surgical repair and placement of a short arm cast. The client reports that the use of the prescribed discharge pain medication (oxycodone 5 mg every 4 hours as needed) is not effective. He currently has 8/10 pain in his right forearm and hand.

VITAL SIGNS

	1430
Temp	98.9 °F oral
HR	105
BP	145/92
RR	22
Pulse oximetry	98% on room air

PHYSICAL ASSESSMENT

Body System	1430
Neurological	Alert and oriented ×4. Conversive. A tingling sensation is present in the right hand.
Pulmonary	Lung sounds are clear. Mildly tachypneic.
Cardiovascular	Heart rate is regular. Trace edema present to the right fingers. Strong left radial pulse. Right radial pulse not accessible for palpation due to cast.
Gastrointestinal	Reports moderate appetite. Last bowel movement this morning.
Genitourinary	Voiding 300 mL cloudy brown urine. The client denies pain with urination.
Integumentary	Skin is dry. Incision on chin is approximated, six stitches intact, mild erythema at incision. Purple bruising present under the eyes bilaterally. Right hand is pale and cool to the touch.
Musculoskeletal	Fiberglass cast in place to right forearm for ulnar fracture. Limited movement of right hand and fingers. 10/10 pain in the right arm and hand.

LABORATORY RESULTS

Laboratory Test and Reference Range	Result, 1430
Sodium Adult: 135–145 mEq/L	138
Potassium Adult: 3.5–5.0 mEq/L	5.4
Calcium Adult: 8.5–10.5 mg/dL	10.9
Creatinine Adult male: 0.6–1.2 mg/dL	1.1
Glucose Adult: 60–100 mg/dL	95
Creatine kinase Adult male: 20–200 U/L	78,000

1. The nurse reviews the assessment data, vital signs, and laboratory values. From the following list, select the assessment findings that require <u>immediate</u> follow up. (Select all that apply)

1. Skin coloration
2. Pain
3. Paresthesia
4. Ecchymosis
5. Urine output
6. Heart rate, 105
7. Respirations, 22
8. Laboratory results

2. The nurse should recognize that the client is <u>most likely</u> experiencing _____ and _____. (Select two answers)

1. deep vein thrombosis
2. compartment syndrome
3. urinary tract infection
4. rhabdomyolysis

<u>NURSES' NOTES (EMERGENCY DEPARTMENT)</u>

Day 1, 1445: The primary physician was notified of the client's condition. The client was diagnosed with compartment syndrome of the right forearm and subsequent rhabdomyolysis per the physician.

3. The nurse reviews the client's diagnoses and recognizes that the client is at risk for several potential complications. From the list below, select the complications for which the client is at the <u>most immediate</u> risk. (Select all that apply)

1. Cardiac arrhythmias
2. Pulmonary embolism
3. Acute renal failure
4. Loss of limb
5. Acute pancreatitis

4. For the following list of potential nursing interventions, specify whether each one is indicated or not indicated.

Potential Nursing Interventions	Indicated	Not Indicated
Apply a cool compress to the client's right hand and arm.	O	O
Apply electrocardiogram patches and attach to the telemetry monitor.	O	O
Elevate the client's right arm to reduce swelling.	O	O
Prepare the client for immediate cast removal.	O	O
Instruct the client to void into a urinal.	O	O

5. The nurse anticipates multiple new orders from the primary care physician. Complete the following sentences with the most appropriate choice from the options given.

The nurse should get ready to administer _____.

1. furosemide 40 mg via IV
2. Dilaudid 0.5 mg via IV
3. ampicillin 1.5 g via IV

It would be a priority for the nurse to infuse _____.

1. 0.9% sodium chloride (normal saline) via IV at 200 mL/hr
2. 5% dextrose in normal saline (D5NS) with 20 mEq potassium chloride (KCl), 500 mL via IV once
3. one unit of packed red blood cells

The nurse should prepare the client for surgery within _____.

1. 2 hours
2. 12 hours
3. 24 hours

Nurses' Notes (Intensive Care Unit)

Day 2, 1200: The client is day 1 status post-emergency fasciotomy to his right arm for suspected compartment syndrome and subsequent rhabdomyolysis. The fasciotomy incision is to remain open until the pressure in the limb has decreased. The right arm is currently immobilized, and the ulnar fracture is stabilized. A patient-controlled analgesia pump is in place with a basal rate of 0.2 mg/hr. The client is awake and alert and is answering questions appropriately. His heart rate is regular, and the telemetry monitor shows normal sinus rhythm. His right hand is pale and cool to the touch. The client reports a mild aching pain of 2/10 intensity in his right arm and hand as well as numbness in his fingertips of the right hand. The client is unable to flex or extend his right wrist or to move the fingers of his right hand.

Vital Signs

	Day 1, 1430	Day 2, 1200
Temp	98.9 °F oral	100.4 °F oral
HR	105	89
BP	145/92	118/76
RR	22	18
Pulse oximetry	98% on room air	96% on room air

6. For the following list of assessment findings, specify whether each one indicates that the client's condition has improved, is unchanged, or has worsened.

Assessment Findings	Improved	Unchanged	Worsened
Heart rate, 89	O	O	O
Temperature, 100.4 °F oral	O	O	O
Fingertip numbness	O	O	O
Pale skin color	O	O	O
Wrist range of motion	O	O	O

Case Study 3

The client is a frail 80-year-old female with a history of end-stage renal failure and controlled hypertension. She has been receiving hemodialysis for over three years, and in the past 6 months she has required an increase of her daily hemodialysis treatment. Despite this increase, the client's symptoms have worsened, requiring frequent hospitalization. The client, accompanied by her daughter, is being seen by the urology team.

NURSES' NOTES

1400: Upon entering the room, the nurse notes that the client is sitting in a chair with a walker at her side. She has +1 pitting edema to her bilateral feet and ankles, which remains unchanged from previous assessments. The patient's weight has decreased by 7 pounds since her last visit 1 month ago, which the patient contributes to a decreased appetite. The client states that she has pain rated at 7/10 in her abdomen, which is no longer responding to current pain medications as ordered. She also reports that she is getting forgetful and often needs breaks while getting ready in the morning or when preparing a meal. Her daughter notes that the client recently has been sleeping more than usual and frequently discusses death, which the daughter finds concerning.

VITAL SIGNS

	1400
Temp	98.9 °F axillary
HR	112
BP	130/78
RR	24
Pulse oximetry	97% on room air

1. In the context of the client's clinical picture, which of the following findings combine to indicate the need for an end-of-life conversation? (Select all that apply)

1. Pain 7/10
2. Decreased appetite
3. +1 pitting edema
4. Increase in sleeping
5. HR 112
6. Frequent discussions of death
7. Daily hemodialysis with worsening symptoms

NURSES' NOTES

1430: The client's status is discussed with the physician, and it is agreed that it is time to consider arranging for additional support for the client and to discuss the possibility of palliative and/or hospice care.

2. When deciding which team(s) to consult, the nurse educates the client and her daughter on the characteristics of the palliative care and hospice care services. Identify whether each of the below supportive services are provided in palliative care, hospice care, or both.

Supportive Services	Palliative Care	Hospice Care	Both
Is provided in conjunction with curative treatment	O	O	O
Prioritizes comfort care	O	O	O
Provides symptom management	O	O	O
Requires a prognosis of ≤6 months	O	O	O
Can be provided during any stage of disease	O	O	O
Provides physical and psychosocial support	O	O	O

NURSES' NOTES

1500: The client voices a desire to stop all treatment because she feels that she spends more time at the dialysis center than in her own home. The physician explains that, should she stop treatment, the disease state will progress, and he offers a prognosis of ≤6 months in this case. The client verbalizes understanding and restates her desire to stop treatment and enroll in hospice care. The physician notes that he will arrange for hospice services and advises on the need for advance directives.

3. Based on the physician's advice regarding advance directives, the nurse must prioritize educating the client on which of the following? (Select all that apply)

1. Living will
2. The appointment of a guardian
3. Do-not-resuscitate (DNR) order
4. Healthcare power of attorney (POA)
5. Promissory note

NURSES' NOTES

1630: After allowing the client and her daughter time to discuss the physician's recommendations, the client and daughter both explain that there is a DNR and living will in place, but when discussing hospice versus palliative care, a disagreement takes place over whether the client should continue treatment despite her noted decline.

4. What is the <u>most</u> appropriate solution by the healthcare team in treating this client?

1. Follow the client's wishes to stop treatment but wait to consult hospice.
2. Follow the daughter's wishes because she is the healthcare POA, and arrange for the next cycle of treatment.
3. Follow the client's wishes to stop treatment and arrange for hospice.
4. Follow the client's and her daughter's wishes by holding treatment for a week and consulting palliative services so the client can continue to receive treatment.

PROGRESS NOTE

Approximately 45 days later, the client has declined drastically and is admitted to an inpatient hospice facility because she stated in her living will that she did not wish to die at home. The home hospice team has determined that death is likely to occur within the next week. The hospice inpatient facility nurse assesses the client after she is settled in to her room. The nurse reports that the client's hands and feet are mottled and retracting, and an audible rattling is heard when the client breathes and coughs. The client is not showing overt signs of pain. The client has lost 3 lb since she was last weighed 1 week ago. The client's daughter reported to the nurse that she ate a full meal within the last 24 hours, although she has refused to eat or drink since, and that the client was able to share that she is at peace with her approaching death.

5. The nurse plans for several interventions to help support the client at the end of her life. For the following list of potential nursing interventions, specify whether each one is indicated or not indicated.

Potential Nursing Interventions	Indicated	Not Indicated
Provide a light massage.	O	O
Administer morphine sulfate 10 mg PO.	O	O
Offer multiple small meals.	O	O
Moisten the client's mouth and lips.	O	O
Reposition the client for comfort every 2 hours.	O	O
Initiate slow continuous IV fluids to minimize the discomfort of thirst.	O	O

6. The daughter notices that her mother is unresponsive and calls out to the nurse for help. The nurse rushes to the client's bedside and determines that the client does not have a pulse. Given the client's signed DNR order, the nurse quietly explains to the daughter that there is nothing left to do. The daughter demands that the medical team initiate cardiopulmonary resuscitation (CPR). When evaluating the client's clinical picture and wishes, what is the nurse's best response?

1. Offer the daughter emotional support and remind her that her mother signed a DNR order, requesting that CPR not be done in this type of circumstance. The team is honoring her mother's wishes.
2. Offer the daughter emotional support and initiate CPR as the daughter has requested because she knows what is best for her mother.
3. Call another nurse to see what he or she thinks should be done.
4. Call the physician for an order to start CPR.

Standalone Questions

1. A patient with interstitial cystitis has been prescribed home bladder instillations with an anesthetic (lidocaine) mixture but has not been doing the instillations consistently because the instillation causes severe burning when she urinates to empty the instillation from the bladder after the prescribed period. Which of the following is likely the best solution?

1. Discontinue the instillations.
2. Clamp the catheter for the prescribed period and then open it to drain the fluid before removal.
3. Remove the catheter after the instillation and then insert a second catheter to drain the bladder.
4. Take an analgesic prior to the instillation.

2. A client tells the nurse that she was recently bitten on the hand by a bat that was inside her house, but the wound has healed. Based on this information, what should the nurse advise the client?

1. No further treatment is necessary.
2. The client must see a physician immediately because the client is at risk for rabies.
3. The client should see a physician because a latent bacterial infection may occur.
4. The client should see the physician if she develops any symptoms.

3. A client has just had a long leg cast applied to his left leg and is in bed. The cast is still damp, and the client is cold. Which of the following actions by the nurse are appropriate? *Select all that apply.*

1. Cover the client, including the cast, with a warm blanket.
2. Cover the client with a warm blanket, leaving the cast exposed to the air.
3. Place a high-powered electric fan to blow directly on the cast.
4. Turn and reposition the client every 2–3 hours.
5. Keep the casted leg elevated whenever possible.

4. Indicate the location of the right lumbar region.

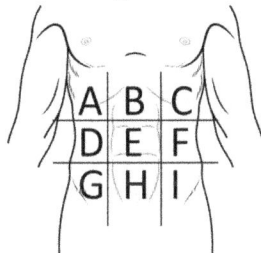

1. A
2. B
3. C
4. D
5. E
6. F
7. G
8. H
9. I

5. A patient with chronic glomerulonephritis has the following nursing diagnoses: activity intolerance, self-care deficit, excess fluid volume, ineffective self-health management, and anxiety. Considering Maslow's hierarchy of needs, which two of these needs should have priority?

1. Excess fluid volume and anxiety
2. Excess fluid volume and self-care deficit
3. Excess fluid volume and activity intolerance
4. Excess fluid volume and ineffective self-health management

6. To facilitate the client's right of autonomy, which of the following assessments by the nurse is the most important?

1. The client's cognitive ability
2. Legal obligations
3. The physician's wishes
4. The client's physical ability

7. A patient has undergone an elective abortion, and according to hospital rules, a nurse who is morally opposed to abortions was excused from caring for the patient. However, the patient's assigned nurse is off of the floor, and as the nurse passes by the patient's room, the patient calls out, "Help, I think I'm bleeding!" Which of the following actions by the nurse is correct?

1. Tell the patient the nurse will find another nurse to examine her.
2. Call the nurse assigned to the patient and ask the nurse to return to examine the patient.
3. Examine the patient for bleeding.
4. Contact a supervisor.

8. A client who has been taking digoxin presents in the emergency department with an irregular pulse, bradycardia of 22–28 bpm, nausea, vomiting, diarrhea, headache, and halo vision. Which of the following interventions should the nurse anticipate? *Select all that apply.*

1. Administer an increased dose of digoxin.
2. Administer digoxin immune fab.
3. Administer atropine.
4. Provide supportive treatment.
5. Conduct laboratory tests for digoxin and electrolyte levels.
6. Carry out continuous cardiac monitoring.

9. When giving an intramuscular injection, which site should the nurse avoid in obese adults?

1. Ventrogluteal
2. Deltoid
3. Dorsogluteal
4. Vastus lateralis

10. A client with Hodgkin's disease has severe pruritus that prevents him from sleeping and causes him considerable discomfort. Which of the following measures may be most effective in relieving itching? *Select all that apply.*

1. Maintaining room humidity at 50–60% and temperature at 70–72 °F
2. Taking diphenhydramine as needed
3. Taking opioid medications
4. Taking oatmeal baths
5. Taking barbiturates

11. The nurse must empty a Hemovac on a postoperative client.

I. Open the plug on the port.
II. Hold the Hemovac over the container and tilt the port toward the container so that fluid drains into the container.
III. Place the plug into the port.
IV. Cleanse the plug and the port with an alcohol wipe in the dominant hand while compressing and holding the top and bottom of the Hemovac together with the other hand.
V. Wash hands and apply gloves.

Place the steps (in Roman numerals) to emptying the Hemovac in the correct order from first to last.

1. _____
2. _____
3. _____
4. _____
5. _____

12. A client has terminal cancer. For months, the client's spouse has been teary and obviously grieving about the impending death, but now that death is imminent, the spouse seems detached and relatively unemotional. Which of the following is the most likely reason for the spouse's reaction?

1. Lack of feelings for the spouse
2. State of emotional shock
3. Dulling of responses because of substance abuse
4. Premature completion of anticipatory grief

13. A client is in cervical traction for a herniated cervical disc. The client complains of increasing pain in the jaw and both ears. Which of the following interventions is most indicated?

1. Provide increased analgesia.
2. Adjust the weights.
3. Correct the head position.
4. Correct the body position.

14. A hospital must be evacuated because of flooding in the area. The nurse is working in the neonatal nursery and has been advised to utilize the Baby Mover Safe Babies Apron to transfer infants. How many infants can be moved in one trip with the apron pockets?

1. Two
2. Three
3. Four
4. Five

15. A client is recovering from placement of an implantable cardioverter-defibrillator (ICD) and suddenly exhibits hypotension with narrowing pulse pressure, pulsus paradoxus, distant heart sounds, restlessness, bulging neck veins, and increasing cyanosis. Which of the following is the most likely cause of these signs and symptoms?

1. A perforation of the ventricle with cardiac tamponade
2. Incorrect positioning of the leads
3. A myocardial infarction
4. Heart failure

16. How much fluid should a patient with an ileostomy be advised to drink each day?

1. 800 mL
2. 1,000 mL
3. 1,500 mL
4. 2,000 mL

17. Two months following allogenic hematopoietic cell transplantation, a client has increasing diarrhea, a red rash over parts of the body, and severe generalized itching; the client's sclerae appear slightly yellow-tinged. Which of the following disorders should the nurse suspect?

1. An allergic response to anti-rejection drugs
2. Acute graft-versus-host disease
3. Liver failure
4. Chronic graft-versus-host disease

18. A pregnant client nearing term is experiencing Braxton Hicks contractions (false labor). Which of the following indications are characteristic of Braxton Hicks contractions? *Select all that apply.*

1. They are associated with dilation of the cervix.
2. They are associated with no dilation of the cervix.
3. Discomfort is felt over the uterine fundus, radiating to the lower abdomen and back.
4. Contractions may become rhythmic.
5. Contractions tend to become longer in duration and occur at closer intervals of time.
6. Contractions may resolve with ambulation or pain medication.

19. A client receiving chemotherapy for breast cancer (stage 2) tells the nurse that she is considering complementary therapy to relieve her almost constant nausea and asks the nurse for advice. Which of the following complementary therapies is most likely to be safe and effective?

1. Acupuncture
2. Therapeutic touch
3. Magnetic therapy
4. Herbal therapies

20. Using the R–R method to calculate the heart rate, what heart rate does this ECG strip represent?

1. 80
2. 88
3. 90
4. 94

21. When changing a colostomy appliance, with which of the following should the skin about the stoma be cleansed after the pouch is removed?

1. Soap and water
2. Alcohol swabs
3. Tap water
4. Baby wipes

22. A client is no longer responding to curative treatments. What is the best approach to initiating a discussion about the referral to palliative and hospice care?

1. "Further treatment is not going to help you."
2. "Would you like to transfer to palliative and hospice care?"
3. "Have you thought about stopping all treatments?"
4. "What do you understand about your options for care?"

23. A hospitalized client calls the nurse into the room and reports that another nurse has been rude to her. Which of the following initial responses by the nurse is most appropriate?

1. "I'm sure the nurse didn't mean to be rude."
2. "The nurse was probably just very busy."
3. "I'm sorry! There's no excuse for a nurse being rude."
4. "I'm so sorry you felt that way. Can you tell me what happened?"

24. The hospital receives news that a train has crashed half a mile away and that a cloud of nonlethal hazardous material has blanketed the area. Which of the following emergency responses should the nurse anticipate?

1. Evacuation
2. Shelter in place
3. Relocation of staff and clients to the interior of building
4. Partial evacuation—children and critically ill only

25. A client has developed signs of tardive dyskinesia with repetitive behavior, including lip smacking and tongue protrusion with choreiform movements of the trunk and extremities. Which of the following medications is most likely the cause of these symptoms?

1. Donepezil HCl
2. Fluoxetine HCl
3. Celecoxib
4. Haloperidol

26. A client brought to the emergency department has been exposed to cold temperatures, and his core body temperature is 34 °C. Which of the following rewarming techniques is most indicated?

1. Cardiopulmonary bypass
2. Warm IV fluid administration
3. Warm peritoneal lavage
4. Forced-air warming blankets

27. A client in the psychiatric unit engages in yelling and name-calling with anger escalating, exhibiting the prodromal syndrome. The nurse is concerned that the client is at risk of self- or other-directed violence. Which of the following is the most appropriate initial intervention?

1. Restrain the client.
2. Offer medication to relax the client.
3. Attempt to talk the client down.
4. Call for additional help.

28. The nurse is caring for a client with severe diarrhea and fecal incontinence from a _Clostridioides difficile_ infection. Which of the following infection control precautions should the nurse expect to implement? *Select all that apply.*

1. Use ≥N95 respirators while caring for the client.
2. Use personal protective equipment (gown and gloves) for all contact with the client.
3. Maintain the client in a private room or >3 feet away from other patients.
4. Wash hands with soap and water rather than alcohol antiseptics.
5. Wear masks for all contact with the client.
6. Avoid sharing electronic thermometers used by the client with other clients.

29. **A client has been diagnosed with end-stage kidney disease and is to begin hemodialysis at an outpatient dialysis center. Which of the following types of access is the best option for most clients?**

1. A venous catheter
2. An AV graft
3. An AV fistula
4. An implanted port

30. **Which of the following are examples of personal protective equipment (PPE)?** *Select all that apply.*

1. Back belts
2. Goggles
3. Personal radiation dosimeters
4. Respirators
5. Gloves

31. **A client's blood pressure is 156/92. What is the pulse pressure in mmHg?** *Record your answer as a whole number.*

_____ mmHg

32. **The nurse believes he observes another nurse taking an opioid medication intended for a client. Which of the following initial actions is the most appropriate?**

1. Confront the nurse taking the client's medication.
2. Notify a supervisor about the observation.
3. Notify the client's physician.
4. Carry out a personal investigation.

33. **What type of tachycardia does the following ECG tracing represent?**

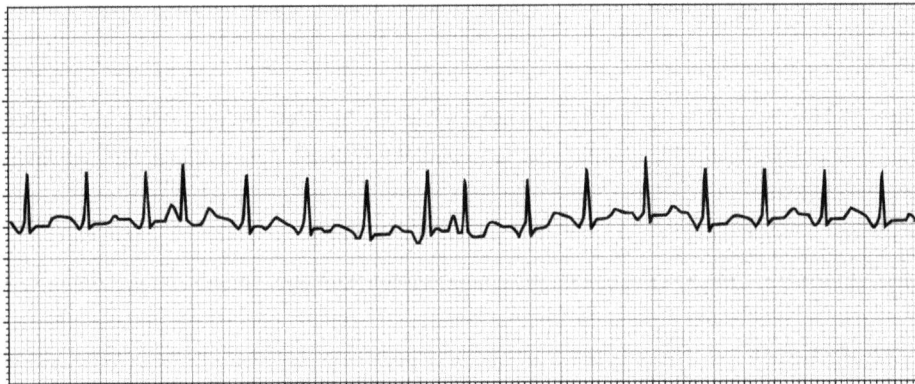

1. Multifocal/multiform atrial tachycardia
2. Junctional tachycardia
3. Sinus tachycardia
4. Torsades de Pointes

34. A client with moderately advanced Alzheimer's disease believes that her deceased husband is living with her and frequently "talks" to him about the happy things they do together. Which is the best nursing response?

1. Tell the client that her husband has died.
2. Try to distract the client when she discusses her husband.
3. Ask the physician for medication to help control the client's hallucinations and delusions.
4. Allow the client to believe that her husband is alive.

35. Which of the following are true regarding premature ventricular contractions? *Select all that apply.*

1. PVCs can be harmless abnormalities.
2. Frequent PVCs signify a myocardial infarction.
3. PVCs can occur in conjunction with underlying dysrhythmias.
4. PVCs can be caused by caffeine, nicotine, or alcohol.

36. A parent tells the nurse that her children, 5 and 10 years old, have been sleeping poorly and complaining of anal itching, occasional abdominal pain, and nausea. What diagnostic test should the nurse anticipate?

1. A complete blood count
2. A tape test
3. An abdominal x-ray
4. A carbon urea breath test

37. The dysrhythmia characterized by a regular heart rate of 150–250 bpm, abnormally shaped P waves (that may be hidden in the preceding T waves), a normal PR interval, and normal QRS complex is:

1. Sinus tachycardia
2. Paroxysmal SVT
3. Junctional dysrhythmia
4. Atrial flutter

38. A client newly diagnosed with schizophrenia has been exhibiting both negative and positive symptoms. Which of the following symptoms would be categorized as negative?

1. Inappropriate affect
2. Visual hallucinations
3. Delusions of grandeur
4. Disheveled appearance

39. A client with diabetes mellitus type 2 is being discharged, and the nurse is instructing the client about safe disposal of syringes and needles at home. Which of the following information should the nurse provide when educating the client? *Select all that apply.*

1. "Place needles and syringes in a sharps disposal container immediately after use."
2. "Keep the container in a safe place out of reach of children and pets."
3. "Dispose of the sharps container in the regular trash can."
4. "Dispose of the sharps container in accordance with community guidelines."
5. "Dispose of the sharps container when it is three-quarters full."
6. "Needles can be flushed down the toilet."

40. The nurse is educating a 23-year-old client about oral contraceptives. Which of the following should the nurse counsel the client to avoid?

1. Drinking alcohol
2. Smoking
3. Eating a high-fat diet
4. Doing aerobic exercises

41. When a client is terminally ill and in the end stages of life, decisions about treatment options, such as whether to provide rehydration, should be based on which of the following considerations?

1. Alleviating symptoms that may cause the family distress
2. Prolonging the client's life as long as possible
3. Following standard protocols for end-of-life care
4. Providing comfort and honoring the client's wishes

42. The rhythm in this ECG strip is best described as:

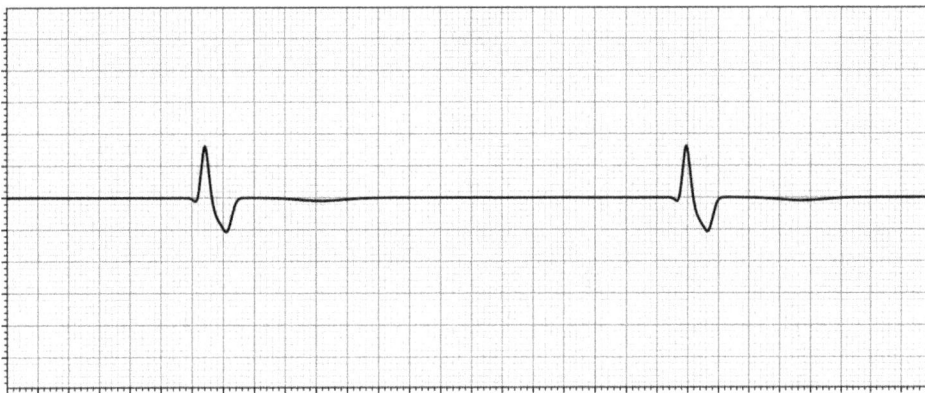

1. Agonal rhythm
2. Pulseless electrical activity
3. Sinus bradycardia
4. Third-degree heart block

43. A 2-year-old child is at the 25th percentile in height but the fourth percentile in weight. The child is slightly anemic, but other laboratory tests, including those for parasites and lead poisoning, are negative. Which of the following is the most likely next step?

1. Identify food allergies and restrictions.
2. Refer the child to Child Protective Services.
3. Observe the child's meal behaviors and practices.
4. Obtain a dietary intake history for the previous 24 hours and the next 3–5 days.

44. Which of the following is the primary purpose in the nurse administering the Apgar (appearance, pulse, grimace, activity, respiration) test to a neonate?

1. To determine the infant's biophysical profile
2. To determine if the infant needs emergency medical care
3. To determine if the infant has congenital defects
4. To determine if the infant is preterm, full term, or post-term

45. A wheelchair-bound client is to be discharged from a rehabilitation facility to the home environment. He still needs minimal assistance for transfers because he is unable to stand and is concerned about transferring from the wheelchair to the toilet and back. Which of the following assistive devices is most indicated to facilitate safe transfer?

1. A gait/transfer belt
2. A full-body sling lift
3. Caregiver assistance only
4. A sliding board

46. The physician has ordered that a client with diabetes insipidus receive 50 mcg of desmopressin acetate by oral tabs twice daily. The tablets are labeled 0.2 mg per tablet. How many tablets will the nurse administer for each dose? *Record your answer as a decimal.*

47. The nurse receives a delivery of a container with this marking (see diagram).

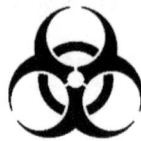

What is the meaning of this international symbol?

1. Poison
2. Medical equipment
3. Biohazard
4. Radioactive

48. A patient has the persistent rhythm shown on the following ECG tracing. What type of rhythm is this?

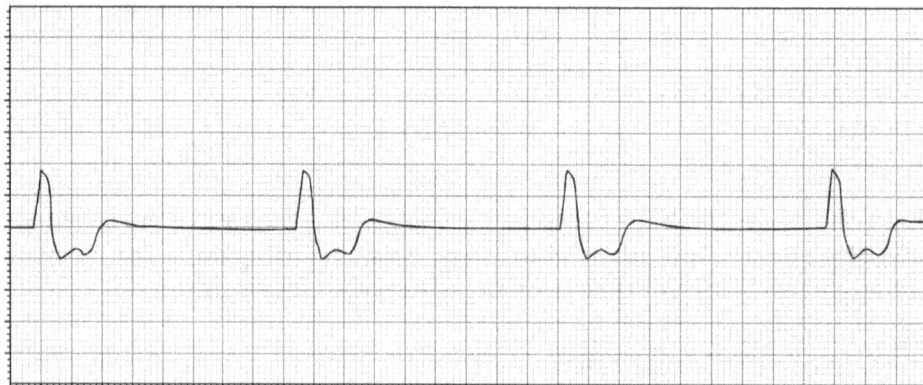

1. Idioventricular rhythm
2. Sinus bradycardia
3. Agonal rhythm
4. Complete (third-degree) heart block

49. A gang member who killed two children in a shooting is hospitalized under police guard and recovering from a gunshot wound. Which of the following violates the ANA Code of Ethics for Nurses?

1. A nurse provides basic care but refuses to talk to the client.
2. A nurse asks to be assigned to a different client.
3. A nurse asks to take vacation time to avoid caring for the client.
4. A nurse tells the team leader that he feels conflicted about caring for the client.

50. Which of the following findings are consistent with early graft rejection in intestine recipients?

1. A change in stool output
2. Decreased hemoglobin and hematocrit
3. Hypotension
4. Decreased serum amylase

51. A client with an inoperable brain tumor is expected to lapse into a coma. Place the usual stages in the continuum of states of consciousness (in Roman numerals) in descending order in the table below:

I. Confusion
II. Delirium
III. Arousal
IV. Vegetative state
V. Stupor

Consciousness
Wakefulness
1. _____
Drowsiness
2. _____
Inattentiveness
3. _____
4. _____
5. _____
Coma

52. A nurse must retrieve supplies on the top shelf of a supply room but cannot reach the shelf, which is about a foot above the nurse's reach. Which of the following is an acceptable work practice?

1. Stand on a footstool.
2. Use a ladder.
3. Climb onto a chair.
4. Step onto the second shelf of the cabinet.

53. The nurse is preparing a mother and neonate for discharge. When educating the parents about infant car seats, which of the following information should the nurse include? *Select all that apply.*

1. "Rear-facing car seats are safer than forward-facing car seats."
2. "Carefully examine a car seat involved in an accident before using again."
3. "The safest positioning of a car seat is in the middle of the back seat."
4. "The neonate's neck should be straight, avoiding the chin-on-chest position."
5. "The harness should be secured until only 3 or 4 fingers slide easily underneath."

54. A client with a long history of alcohol abuse has been prescribed disulfiram so that he will stop drinking. When educating the client about the acetaldehyde syndrome, which of the following effects of combining the drug and alcohol should the nurse include? *Select all that apply.*

1. Nausea and copious vomiting
2. Severe flushing, headache, and vertigo
3. Hypotension, chest pain, and syncope
4. Somnolence progressing to coma

55. Nurse A notes that Nurse B on the unit smells of alcohol and is slightly slurring her words. What is the best course of action for Nurse A?

1. Tell Nurse B that she needs to go home because she appears to be inebriated.
2. Immediately notify a supervisor.
3. Observe Nurse B to ensure that she is providing safe care.
4. Assist Nurse B in caring for her clients until she is less impaired.

56. Following surgical removal of an ovarian cyst, a client has not urinated in 4 hours and feels the urge to urinate but is unable to initiate urine flow. Which of the following should the nurse do initially to promote urination? *Select all that apply.*

1. Pour warm water over the client's perineum while she is on the toilet.
2. Ask the client to blow bubbles through a straw into a glass of water while trying to urinate.
3. Turn on running water while the client tries to urinate.
4. Tell the client to "just relax."
5. Catheterize the client.

57. A client with 2+ peripheral edema and increasing complaints of lethargy has the following laboratory results:

Test	Result
BUN	172 mg/dL
Serum creatinine	16.4 mg/dL
Glucose	98 mg/dL

Which further testing should the nurse expect based on these findings?

1. Testing for diabetes
2. Testing for liver disease
3. Testing for heart disease
4. Testing for kidney disease

58. The nurse has inserted a Foley catheter into a male client who is bedridden. Which of the following is the best position in which to secure the catheter?

1. The penis is positioned down with the Foley catheter taped to the front of the inner thigh, and then the tubing is looped to allow for turning and it is taped to the edge of the bed.
2. The penis is positioned up with the Foley catheter taped to the right or left lower abdomen, and then the tubing is looped to allow for turning and it is taped to the edge of the bed.
3. The penis is left unpositioned with the catheter curved over one leg, and the tubing is looped and secured only to the edge of the bed.
4. The penis is positioned downward with the catheter secured to the posterior thigh, and the tubing is looped and secured to the edge of the bed.

59. When assessing a client's health history regarding intake of alcohol, which of the following would qualify the person as an "at-risk" drinker?

1. A male client who goes out with friends 1 or 2 times a week and has 4–6 drinks
2. A female client who rarely drinks but "got drunk" at a college party 4 years earlier
3. A male client who typically has 2 glasses of wine each day
4. A female client who typically has 5–6 beers per week

60. When assessing the fetal heart rate with the nonstress test (NST) at 34 weeks, what type of accelerations should normally occur during a 20-minute period of observation?

1. At least 2 accelerations of at least 20 bpm over 20 seconds
2. At least 2 accelerations of at least 15 bpm over 15 seconds
3. At least 1 acceleration of at least 10 bpm over 10 seconds
4. At least 1 acceleration of at least 5 bpm over 5 seconds

61. The nurse is educating the parents of a severely allergic child about methods of controlling dust mites. Which of the following actions should the nurse advise the parents are essential? *Select all that apply.*

1. Keep the house clean and free of obvious dust and clutter.
2. Encase the child's mattress and box spring in allergen-proof covers.
3. Remove all carpets from the house.
4. Replace all upholstered furniture with leather or vinyl furniture.
5. Wash bed linens, pillows, clothing, and stuffed toys in hot water once a week.
6. Maintain humidity below 50%.

62. A mother's amniotic fluid is meconium stained. Which of the following complications is the neonate at risk of developing?

1. Anemia
2. Respiratory distress
3. Growth retardation
4. Cognitive impairment

63. Which of the following are age-related changes that typically occur in the respiratory system? *Select all that apply.*

1. Blunting of cough/laryngeal reflexes
2. Fewer alveoli
3. Decreased ciliary action
4. Smaller alveoli
5. Increased elasticity of lung tissue
6. Increased rigidity of thoracic muscles

64. A client has been taking 112 mcg of levothyroxine daily, but the physician has changed the dosage to 0.224 mg daily, and the patient wants to use up the tablets on hand. How many 112 mcg tablets equal 0.224 mg? *Record your answer as a whole number.*

_____ tablets

65. If the nurse is to give a client two oral medications (capsules) per the enteral feeding tube, which of the following is the correct procedure?

1. Open the capsules directly into the feeding formula and instill.
2. Open the capsules together and dilute with water before instilling.
3. Open the capsules separately and dilute each with water before instilling.
4. Oral medications cannot be given per the enteral feeding tube.

66. The nurse is administering an intermittent tube feeding to a client per an NG tube. The nurse has checked the placement of the tube, checked for gastric residual, and aspirated 150 mL of gastric contents. Which of the following next actions is most appropriate?

1. Hold feeding and notify MD of gastric residual.
2. Proceed with tube feeding.
3. Return the aspirated gastric contents to the stomach and flush the tubing with 30 mL water.
4. Return 100 mL of aspirated gastric contents to the stomach followed by the tube feeding.

67. The type of pacemaker malfunction that the following ECG demonstrates is:

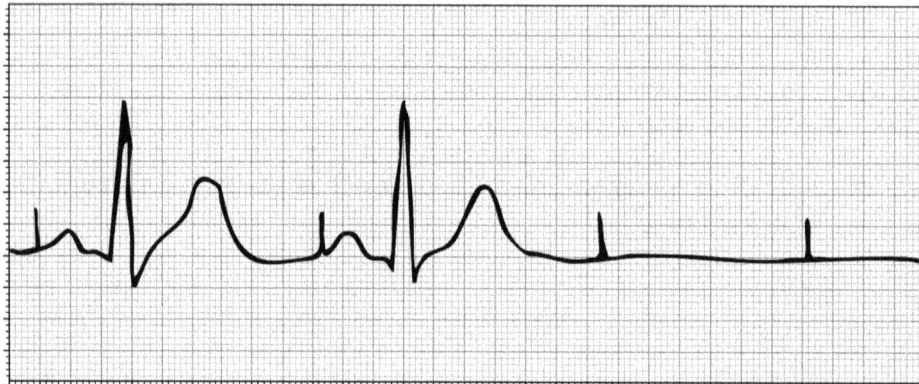

1. No malfunction
2. Failure to sense
3. Failure to capture
4. Failure to pace

68. A patient presents in a deep coma with decorticate posturing, which suggests damage to which part of the brain?

1. Midbrain
2. Right and left hemispheres
3. Medulla
4. Diencephalon

69. When assessing a neonate 's respiratory status, which of the following is an indication of respiratory distress. *Select all that apply.*

1. Respiratory rate of 50 breaths per minute at rest
2. Flaring nostrils
3. Grunting expirations
4. Sternal retraction
5. Intercostal retractions

70. A client is to receive 125 mg of meperidine stat. A vial of meperidine contains 50 mg/mL. How many mL are required to provide a dosage of 125 mg? *Record your answer using one decimal place.*

_____ mL

71. The nurse is caring for a client who is awaiting open reduction and internal fixation (ORIF) of a hip fracture and is temporarily immobilized with Buck's traction. The nurse notes that the knot of the rope is lodged against the pulley. What is the primary concern with this finding?

1. There is no concern because this is the correct placement of the knot.
2. This may change body alignment.
3. This may interfere with the line of pull.
4. This may change the direction of pull.

72. A client at a family planning clinic has received a prescription for oral contraceptives. When reviewing the client's medication list, the nurse notes that the client takes the following:

- St. John's wort 300 mg three times daily
- Vitamin D3 500 mg daily
- Calcium carbonate 1000 mg daily
- Acetaminophen 650 mg every 6 hours as needed for headache
- Multivitamin capsule daily

Which of the following information should the nurse include when educating the client about taking oral contraceptives?

1. These medications and supplements should not interfere with oral contraceptives.
2. Vitamin D3 and calcium carbonate should not be taken with oral contraceptives.
3. St. John's wort may decrease the effectiveness of oral contraceptives.
4. St. John's wort should not be taken with calcium carbonate or multivitamins.

73. Which of the following ensures minimal proper identification prior to administering medication?

1. The nurse recognizes client.
2. The nurse asks the client's name and checks their hospital ID bracelet.
3. The nurse reads the client's name on the intake and output record at the foot of the client's bed.
4. The nurse asks for the client's name.

74. A 15-month-old child who weighs 10 kg is being treated with amoxicillin oral suspension at the rate of 25 mg/kg/day in two divided doses 12 hours apart. How many mg should the child receive at each dose? *Record your answer as a whole number.*

_____ mg

75. A client with kidney failure is considering continuous ambulatory peritoneal dialysis (CAPD). The client asks the nurse for information about CAPD. Which of the following information should the nurse include? *Select all that apply.*

1. Exchanges are usually done with about 2 L of dialysate.
2. Most clients do 4–5 exchanges in a 24-hour period.
3. Each exchange takes 30–40 minutes.
4. An exchange is a clean rather than sterile procedure.
5. Exchanges at night involve a longer period of retention.

76. A 76-year-old female tells the nurse that she and her husband want to continue to engage in sexual activity, but both have osteoarthritis and limited mobility. Which position should the nurse recommend to put the least amount of strain on both partners?

1. "Missionary" position (male on top)
2. Female on top
3. "Spooning" position with male behind female, side-lying
4. Rear vaginal entry with female prone and male on top

77. An adult client has instilled drops into the ear to soften cerumen, and the nurse is to irrigate the ear to remove the cerumen. Which of the following statements are correct about ear irrigations? *Select all that apply.*

1. 50 mL of irrigant should be instilled rapidly to dislodge the cerumen.
2. The tip of the syringe should be used to occlude the ear canal.
3. The pinna should be pulled up and back.
4. Allow fluid to drain out during the procedure.
5. Position client in sitting or lying position.
6. Ask client to turn the head away from the affected ear.

78. The nurse is working as a team leader and discussing assignments with team members. Which of the following statements to the group by a team member is a HIPAA violation of privacy?

1. "Mrs. Brown says she has no support system when she goes home."
2. "Mrs. Brown says she has been having an affair with her husband's brother!"
3. "Mrs. Brown says she dislikes her therapist, so she refuses to cooperate."
4. "Mrs. Brown seems angry all of the time and yells at her family when they visit."

79. The nurse is documenting the interview with a client with asthma and diabetes. Which of the following documentations is correct? *Select all that apply.*

1. "Client appears SOB and anxious."
2. "Client took a nebulizer treatment with .25 mg budesonide inhalation suspension prior to visit."
3. "Client needs new a prescription for 0.5% albuterol inhalation solution."
4. "Client checks their blood sugar Q.O.D."
5. "Client exhibits dyspnea and tachypnea (26/min)."

80. The nurse must administer 5 mL of acetaminophen solution through the nasogastric (NG) tube of a client, but the NG tube is attached to suction. How long (in minutes) should the nurse discontinue the suction after administering the medication? *Record your answer as a whole number.*

_____ minutes

81. The nurse is caring for four clients, all of whom need attention:

I. A 6-hour postoperative client is asking for pain medication for pain of 8 on a scale of 1–10.
II. A 2-day postoperative client needs a routine dressing change.
III. A 5-day postoperative client needs intermittent tube feeding.
IV. A 3-day postoperative client needs assessment for sudden elevated temperature.

Prioritize the clients (in Roman numerals) according to the order in which the nurse should attend to them.

1. ____
2. ____
3. ____
4. ____

82. A client has undergone gastric bypass surgery but is experiencing severe dumping syndrome after eating. Which of the following should the nurse advise the client to avoid? *Select all that apply.*

1. Concentrated sugars
2. Fluids with meals
3. Whole milk and yogurt
4. Reclining after eating
5. Large meals

83. A pregnant client is at term and in the first stages of labor, and the nurse is monitoring the fetal heart rate. Which of the following is the normal fetal heart rate at term?

1. 60–90 bpm
2. 90–100 bpm
3. 120–160 bpm
4. 160–200 bpm

84. The nurse is caring for an elderly client who had a severe myocardial infarction and whose death appears imminent. Even though healthcare providers are still trying to save the client's life, family members are insisting that she be dressed in her culture's traditional clothing that they have brought from home. Which of the following is the most appropriate response?

1. Tell them that they cannot interrupt treatment.
2. Suggest they wait until efforts to save the client end.
3. Assist them to dress the client if possible.
4. Advise them that clothing is not important.

85. The nurse must give an intramuscular injection to an adult. What length of needle is most appropriate?

1. 0.5–0.75 in
2. 0.75–1.0 in
3. 1.0–1.5 in
4. 1.5–2.0 in

86. A pregnant client tells the nurse that she is Rh– and her husband is Rh+, but she believes she does not need to receive RhoGAM with a first pregnancy. Which of the following is the best response?

1. "You are right, but you will need the treatment during a second pregnancy."
2. "You need treatment during your first pregnancy to prevent Rh incompatibility reactions during a second pregnancy."
3. "You are wrong. You need the treatment with your first pregnancy."
4. "You should ask the doctor about that."

87. Which of the following is a common psychosocial response of a pregnant client to pregnancy during the first trimester?

1. Increasing dependency
2. Alteration in body image
3. Ambivalence
4. Changes in sexuality

88. A client tells the nurse that he wants to designate his son to make only his healthcare decisions in the event that he is not able to do so, but he is unsure what document he needs to complete. Which of the following should the nurse advise?

1. A living will
2. An advance directive
3. A power of attorney
4. A durable power of attorney for healthcare

89. Following an automobile accident that resulted in what appeared to be a mild head injury and fractured right clavicle, the client is being carefully monitored. The client's telemetry had shown a normal ECG complex with a normal pulse rate until the following changes occurred:

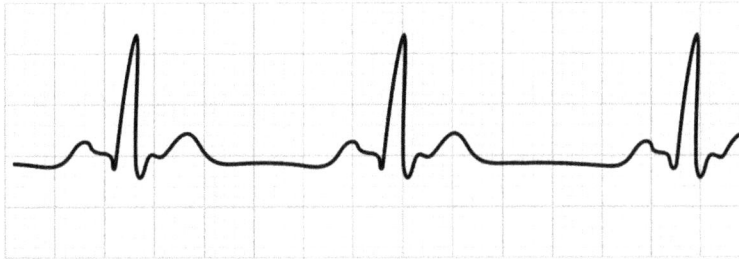

What does this tracing most likely represent?
1. Sinus bradycardia resulting from increasing intracranial pressure
2. Sinus bradycardia resulting from hypovolemia
3. Premature ventricular contraction resulting from hypovolemia
4. Premature ventricular contraction resulting from increasing intracranial pressure

90. If a client is walking in the hall and falls to the floor with a tonic-clonic seizure, which of the following actions by the nurse is the most appropriate. *Select all that apply.*
1. Turn the client to one side with their head slightly flexed forward.
2. Restrain the client to prevent injury.
3. Insert a padded tongue blade between the teeth if possible.
4. Support the head with cushioning of some type.
5. Provide privacy if possible.

91. A client has been diagnosed with amyotrophic lateral sclerosis (ALS) and uses a wheelchair but still breathes independently. At what point may the client receive palliative care?
1. When the client becomes ventilator dependent or near death
2. When the client's life expectancy is 6 months or less
3. At any time since the client has a life-threatening disease
4. When the client is in need of pain control

92. An ECG exam is being performed on a patient with suspected pacemaker malfunction. What does the following tracing suggest?

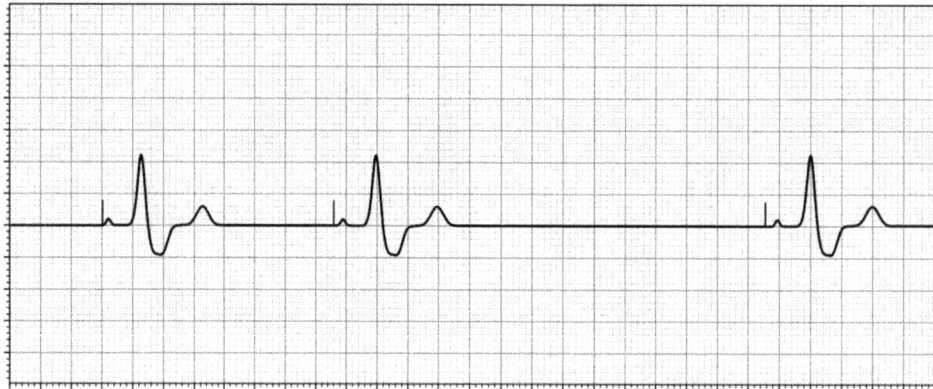

1. Failure to sense
2. Normal functioning
3. Failure to capture
4. Failure to pace

93. The nurse is working in the emergency department. Which of the following injuries must be reported to the police or appropriate authorities?

1. A woman has multiple facial injuries and defensive wounds on her hands and arms, but she insists she fell.
2. A 6-year-old child has severe head and face injuries and multiple broken ribs. X-rays indicate numerous old orthopedic injuries, and the mother states the child fell off a swing.
3. A client has a large open cut on his torso and claims he was injured when a large light fixture fell on him.
4. An 18-year-old girl who was severely intoxicated from drinking fell and broke her arm.

94. The nurse has obtained a unit of packed red blood cells that is to be administered to a client with leukemia. Within how many minutes must the transfusion be initiated after removal from the blood bank refrigerator?

1. 15 minutes
2. 30 minutes
3. 45 minutes
4. 60 minutes

95. An infant is to receive 65 mg of acetaminophen elixir every 4–6 hours as needed for fever. The elixir contains 80 mg per 5 mL. How many mL should be administered to equal 65 mg? *Record your answer rounding to the nearest whole number.*

_____ mL.

96. The nurse is discussing the use of condoms with a 19-year-old male. Which of the following information should the nurse include about latex condom use? *Select all that apply.*

1. Latex condoms should be used with nonoxynol-9.
2. Latex condoms should be used for every act of oral, vaginal, and anal sex.
3. Oil-based lubricants may be used with latex condoms.
4. Condoms should be removed immediately after ejaculation before the penis becomes flaccid.
5. A condom may be left in place and used for two acts of sex if the acts occur within 30 minutes of each other.
6. Condoms provide 100% protection against pregnancy, human immunodeficiency virus (HIV), and sexually transmitted diseases (STDs).

97. A client is receiving warfarin for venous thrombosis, and the client's INR is 4.0 with no evidence of bleeding. What action does the nurse anticipate?

1. Administer warfarin as prescribed.
2. Administer increased dosage of warfarin until INR increases.
3. Hold or administer reduced dosage until INR decreases.
4. Hold warfarin and administer vitamin K orally.

98. A client receiving treatment for breast cancer feels severely anxious. Which of the following interventions are likely to be the most effective? *Select all that apply.*

1. Instructing the client in relaxation exercises
2. Encouraging the client to express concerns
3. Advising the client that the anxiety will reduce in time
4. Reminding the client that recovery rates are high
5. Determining what relieves the client's anxiety

99. Which metabolic effect is most common if a client is taking a loop diuretic?

1. Hypouricemia
2. Hyperglycemia
3. Hyperkalemia
4. Hypokalemia

100. The first indication of amniotic fluid embolism (also called pregnancy-related anaphylactoid syndrome) is usually sudden onset of which of the following?

1. Severe chest pain
2. Acute dyspnea
3. Hemorrhage
4. Hypotension

Answer Key and Explanations for Test #3

Case Study 1

1. 3, 5, and 6: The client's integumentary assessment results require attention because he has multiple sites of entry for bacteria. The laceration near his deformity is especially concerning because this is a potential route for infection to enter the bone. The client's musculoskeletal assessment is notable because it shows signs of damage to the wrist and/or hand. Further diagnostics will be required to verify the extent of the injury. The mechanism of injury is important information to have for any traumatic injury because it can assist the healthcare team in assessing the likely severity of an injury and what resources may be required to treat the client. The fact that the client was not wearing safety gear should also be noted because this increases his risk of a more severe injury. The client's blood pressure, heart rate, and tachypnea (as evidenced by the pulmonary assessment) should certainly be noted as elevated, but, given the other assessment data, these are likely caused by increased stress from the client's level of pain. If these remain elevated after the pain is treated and the client's stress is reduced, further assessment should be conducted to find the underlying cause.

2. 3: Given the mechanism of injury, laceration to the wrist, the decreased range of motion, and deformity to the wrist, this client is most likely experiencing an open fracture. Dislocation could be possible as well (and it should be ruled out), but because the client fell and landed on his wrist, there is more likely a fracture from the impact than a dislocation (which is typically caused by a pulling mechanism to the joint). Compartment syndrome is a concern, as swelling to the wrist causes an increased risk for this complication, but this is not a likely diagnosis because the client's pain is relieved with analgesics, pulses are present distal to the injury, and the client denies any tingling of his fingers. Osteomyelitis is the least likely complication because the injury just occurred and it takes time for a bone infection to set in. However, it would be important to consider this complication in the context of older open injuries.

3.

- Administer IV cefazolin.
- Obtain urine toxicology results.
- Administer the tetanus, diphtheria, and pertussis (Tdap) vaccine.
- Obtain blood work.
- Obtain an x-ray of the affected limb.
- Educate the client on skateboard safety.

When an open fracture is suspected, the most important initial interventions are to administer a prophylactic antibiotic (in this case, cefazolin) and obtain imaging to confirm the extent of the injury. The antibiotic should be given as soon as possible to prevent the risk of osteomyelitis or other infection to the wound. Also, the sooner an x-ray is performed, the sooner the injury can be diagnosed so that further interventions (such as a reduction) can be performed early to preserve the integrity of the limb, reducing the risk of impaired circulation in the extremity and poor healing to the bone. Although, in many cases, obtaining blood work is among the top priorities to diagnose medical conditions, it is not as useful in the majority of relatively minor traumatic orthopedic injuries. This client does not currently have signs of infection or significant blood loss, so blood work is useful simply as a preliminary assessment if the client needed emergent surgery. Administration of the Tdap vaccine is important in this client because his open wound increases his

132

risk of tetanus. However, it can be administered after the client is fully assessed and stabilized because tetanus is unlikely to set in for several days (if at all). It is important to educate the client on skateboard safety, but this is not the priority at this time and would likely be inappropriate while the client is still in a lot of pain, has not been diagnosed or treated yet, and is likely under a lot of stress. This information is more appropriate to discuss after the client's condition has been treated and would go well with discharge education.

4.

Potential Nursing Interventions	Indicated	Not Indicated
Place the client on cardiac and capnography monitoring.	●	○
Prepare for intubation.	○	●
Anticipate the administration of an IV fluid bolus.	●	○
Set up bedside suction and bag valve mask.	●	○
Start a second IV on the left forearm.	○	●

Administration of procedural sedation (especially with medications such as Propofol) can cause hypotension and respiratory depression. The best way to monitor for respiratory depression is with capnography. An IV fluid bolus should be ready for use in case it is needed to treat hypotension. Bedside suction and a bag valve mask should be nearby in case the client's airway becomes compromised during sedation. Although there should be resuscitation supplies (including an intubation tray) nearby in case of an adverse event during the client's sedation, intubation is not anticipated in this form of IV procedural sedation, in which it is only deep enough to blunt pain and relax the extremity. The client should be able to maintain his own airway. Although a second IV may be useful, it should not be started on the injured limb because it will likely be covered by the splint.

5. 2, 3, and 5: The client's vitals show that he is likely having the common reactions to Propofol of respiratory depression and hypotension. The initial interventions to treat these are to administer supplemental oxygen, open the airway using the jaw thrust maneuver, and administer an IV fluid bolus. IV naloxone is not indicated because Propofol is not an opiate and naloxone would have no effect. The client had received an opiate (fentanyl), but it was given more than 1 hour prior to this event and is unlikely to be the cause of the respiratory depression and hypotension. The client does not appear to be having an anaphylactic reaction; therefore, epinephrine is not indicated at this time. The client currently has a pulse, so CPR is not indicated. However, if his respiratory depression and hypotension were not reversed successfully, he could progress into cardiac arrest and require CPR.

6. 2, 3, and 6: Clients who are discharged from the hospital with fractures should be referred to an orthopedic specialist. The client was placed in a temporary splint in the emergency department and may need a cast and/or surgical repair depending on the orthopedic specialist's assessment. Casts should not be placed immediately after an injury in the emergency department because swelling of the affected limb is likely to increase in the coming days. Splints can be adjusted around this swelling to reduce the risk of compartment syndrome. Casts are solid and cannot be adjusted without being fully removed. The client should return to the emergency department if his pain is so severe that prescribed pain medications do not help, as this may be a sign of compartment syndrome. Additionally, the client should know that if his fingers become painful or numb, he should loosen the elastic bandage of his splint to prevent compartment syndrome. He should also be instructed that he should return if loosening the bandage does not improve the pain or numbness. The client is correct that the maximum dose of acetaminophen for an adult is 4,000 mg in 1 day. This should be emphasized with clients who are prescribed analgesics that include a combination of an opiate and acetaminophen. If it is safe for the client to take them, nonsteroidal anti-inflammatory agents can also be encouraged for pain relief because they help with inflammation. If the client notices that he has a fever or purulent drainage, he should return to the emergency department because this is a sign of infection of his wound. Finally, the client does not need to wear his sling for the first 24 hours or when he sleeps. This would more likely be an instruction for a client with a shoulder dislocation. In ulnar fractures, slings are mainly used to promote comfort and decrease the use of the limb during the healing process.

Case Study 2

1. 1, 2, 3, 5, and 8: The client has several symptoms indicating potentially poor perfusion to his right arm, including skin pallor, pain, and paresthesia. The client's dark urine color is abnormal and should be followed up on. The client also has multiple laboratory results that are outside the normal limits. Although facial bruising can be concerning, it would be expected with a history of a recent nasal fracture and would not require immediate follow-up. Although the heart rate and respirations should be monitored closely, it is not unusual for these to be mildly elevated in the setting of severe pain.

2. 2 and 4: The client is demonstrating three signs of compartment syndrome in his right extremity: extreme pain, pallor, and paresthesia. Because the client also has two known risk factors (recent fracture and a cast in place), the nurse should suspect compartment syndrome. Rhabdomyolysis is a potential complication of compartment syndrome as the muscle cells are destroyed and release their contents into the bloodstream. This can cause severely elevated creatine kinase levels as well as elevated serum potassium and calcium. Dark-brown-colored urine is considered a hallmark sign of rhabdomyolysis and is usually due to the presence of myoglobin in the urine as a result of muscle breakdown. Although a deep vein thrombosis also can cause swelling and pain, it typically results in skin that is warm to the touch and red in appearance in the affected extremity. Although a urinary tract infection can also result in dark-colored urine, there are no other symptoms present at this time making it less likely in this situation.

3. 1, 3, and 4: The client is at risk for cardiac arrhythmias due to elevated potassium and calcium levels present. Elevated creatine kinase levels in the blood can severely damage the kidneys and potentially lead to acute renal failure. The client is also at risk for needing a limb amputation if the compartment syndrome is not addressed and relieved. The client is not at immediate risk for a pulmonary embolism because there is no sign of a blood clot at this time. The client does not currently have common risk factors for acute pancreatitis (such as elevated triglycerides, excessive alcohol consumption, or gallstones).

4.

Potential Nursing Interventions	Indicated	Not Indicated
Apply a cool compress to the client's right hand and arm.	○	●
Apply electrocardiogram patches and attach to the telemetry monitor.	●	○
Elevate the client's right arm to reduce swelling.	○	●
Prepare the client for immediate cast removal.	●	○
Instruct the client to void into a urinal.	●	○

Due to the electrolyte shifts present with rhabdomyolysis, the client is at a high risk for cardiac arrhythmias, so continuous telemetry monitoring would be indicated. In order to reduce external compression on the arm, the client's cast would need to be removed as soon as possible. The nurse should also educate the client to use a urinal so that his urine can be monitored and assessed because the client is at risk for acute kidney injury due to rhabdomyolysis. With compartment syndrome, the nurse should not apply cool compresses due to the resulting vasoconstriction and further restriction of blood flow to the arm. Similarly, the nurse should not elevate the affected extremity because this would also reduce perfusion of his arm.

5. First drop-down: 2. The client is in severe pain, and the nurse should anticipate orders to address his pain with a strong analgesic. Furosemide may be used if the client does not produce adequate urine, but it would not be needed at this time because the client is voiding adequately. There is no sign of infection at this time, so ampicillin would not be indicated. **Second drop-down: 1.** With rhabdomyolysis, isotonic IV fluids such as normal saline help prevent kidney damage by diluting myoglobin in the blood. D5NS with 20 mEq KCl would not be appropriate for the client at this time because he already has an elevated potassium level. There is no indication for a blood transfusion at this time. **Third drop-down: 1.** Compartment syndrome is a medical emergency, and the client would need emergency surgery in order to prevent permanent damage to his arm. The nurse should prepare the client for surgery as soon as possible.

6.

Assessment Findings	Improved	Unchanged	Worsened
Heart rate, 89	●	○	○
Temperature, 100.4 °F oral	○	○	●
Fingertip numbness	○	○	●
Pale skin color	○	●	○
Wrist range of motion	○	○	●

The client's heart rate is lower than at admission, which may be a result of better pain control with the patient-controlled analgesia pump. His temperature is higher than at admission, which could be an early sign of infection, which the client is at high risk for due to having an open wound following the fasciotomy. The client has possible worsening compartment syndrome because the fingertip tingling present on admission has now progressed to numbness. The pale skin color, although still being indicative of compartment syndrome, is unchanged from admission. The client's inability to move the affected wrist is of concern for paralysis—a late symptom of compartment syndrome and often indicative of irreversible muscle damage.

Case Study 3

1. 2, 4, 6, and 7: Although any discussion surrounding end-of-life care has varied indications, this client is demonstrating a declining status despite increased interventions. Because this client has end-stage renal disease that is no longer responding to daily hemodialysis treatments, the prognosis is grave. This—combined with a decrease in appetite, increases in sleeping/napping, and a new focus on death—warrants a conversation about end-of-life concerns with regard to the client's understanding and wishes. These signs indicate the client's body and mind are preparing for the dying process. The client's pain is not new but requires frequent assessment to determine new treatment options. The client's edema is not new either. The tachycardia may be reflective of the client's pain level and should be monitored.

2.

Supportive Services	Palliative Care	Hospice Care	Both
Is provided in conjunction with curative treatment	●	○	○
Prioritizes comfort care	○	○	●
Provides symptom management	○	○	●
Requires a prognosis of ≤6 months	○	●	○
Can be provided during any stage of disease	●	○	○
Provides physical and psychosocial support	○	○	●

Palliative care and hospice care services both offer physical and mental support and treatment in addition to symptom management. Hospice requires a prognosis of ≤6 months and an end to efforts at curative treatment. Palliative care provides support for clients during any stage of their disease process and can be provided concurrently with active treatment. Palliative care is often consulted when a client has multiple symptoms that require frequent evaluation for management, allowing the disease team to focus on treating the primary illness.

3. 1, 3, and 4: The nurse must prioritize educating the client and her family on the formal documents that fall under the category of advance directives per the physician's advice. A living will, do-not-resuscitate (DNR) order, and healthcare power of attorney (POA) are legal designations that allow the client to state her wishes regarding medical interventions and end-of-life care in case she no longer has the capacity to make these decisions as her disease progresses. The healthcare POA allows the client to name an individual to make medical decisions on his or her behalf when incapacitated, if not already outlined in the DNR or living will. Appointment of a guardian and a promissory note are also legal designations that are not related to the client's wishes relating to end-of-life issues. The appointment of a guardian is done when an individual is deemed incapacitated or is unable to make his or her own decisions, usually related to property or finances. A promissory note is an agreement to pay back a loan.

4. 3: Despite some forgetfulness, the client remains of sound mind, and she has clearly expressed her wishes regarding her care plan. The medical team must identify what the client's wishes are and ensure that the care plan meets these expectations, specifically those outlined in a DNR and living will. In this case, curative treatment should cease and hospice is arranged. The client's healthcare POA would not be indicated to make decisions for the client at this time because she is mentally capable to do so herself. All of the other options violate these legal documents and leave the team open to litigation.

5.

Potential Nursing Interventions	Indicated	Not Indicated
Provide a light massage.	●	○
Administer morphine sulfate 10 mg PO.	○	●
Offer multiple small meals.	○	●
Moisten the client's mouth and lips.	●	○
Reposition the client for comfort every 2 hours.	●	○
Initiate slow continuous IV fluids to minimize the discomfort of thirst.	○	●

Given that the client is showing signs of contractures, or tightening of the muscles, the nurse can provide light massage to help ease the discomfort associated with this end-of-life process. Keeping the client's mouth and lips moist provides comfort, without providing enough fluids to prolong the dying process (which would occur if the client was administered IV fluids). Repositioning the client allows for comfort and ensures that skin breakdown does not occur. If extreme pain was induced when repositioning the client, this would no longer be indicated. Pain medication by mouth (PO) is not indicated because the client is not demonstrating pain and likely would not tolerate PO medication at this time. The client has refused nutrition, which is a sign that her body is preparing for death; therefore, even small meals are not needed.

6. 1: A signed DNR is a legally binding document; therefore, the nurse's best course of action is to abide by the wishes outlined in the document and withhold any life-sustaining measures, including CPR. She should also provide the daughter with the emotional support needed during this difficult time. Calling another nurse or the physician is not indicated because the nurse must follow the DNR order as written regardless of her own personal opinion, and this would divert attention from supporting the daughter, which is the priority at this time.

Standalone Questions

1. 2: The best solution for the interstitial cystitis patient who experiences severe burning when emptying the bladder after an instillation is to leave the catheter in place, clamp it for the prescribed period, and then open the catheter to drain the solution. If the patient finds the catheter itself irritating, it can be removed and replaced with a second catheter to drain the bladder, but a better solution is to try to change the type or size of the catheter to find one that is less irritating.

2. 2: The client must see a physician immediately because she is at risk for rabies; most cases of rabies in the United States are traced to infections from bats. Most bats that humans are able to approach are ill, increasing the danger. Rabies prophylaxis must be given before the onset of neurological symptoms, so the nurse should stress that the client should not wait to see if symptoms occur because once she develops rabies, death is almost certain.

3. 2, 4, 5: The nurse should cover the client with a warm blanket, leaving the cast exposed to the air so that it can dry properly. The client should be turned and repositioned every 2–3 hours so that all sides of the cast can dry evenly, while also keeping the casted leg elevated whenever possible to minimize swelling. While some facilities use heat cradles or commercial cast dryers at low temperatures, high-powered electric fans should not blow directly on the cast as this may result in the outside drying and the inside remaining damp.

4. 4:

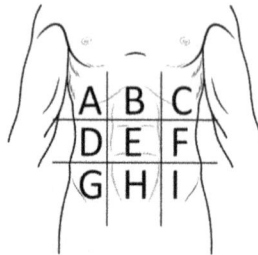

A. Right hypochondriac
B. Epigastric
C. Left hypochondriac
D. Right lumbar
E. Umbilical
F. Left lumbar
G. Right Inguinal
H. Hypogastric/Suprapubic
I. Left Inguinal

5. 1: The first need that should be addressed is the excess fluid volume because it is a physiological need. Physiological needs should always be dealt with first. The second need to consider is the anxiety because it is a safety need, which involves the need for security and to be free of fear and anxiety.

6. 1: The ethical principle of autonomy recognizes that clients have the right to make their own informed decisions about their care. The most important assessment is of the client's cognitive ability because the client needs to be able to understand and consider information that is given by healthcare providers. Children may be able to make informed decisions, but the law does not allow them to do so unless they are emancipated, so the right of autonomy passes to the parents or guardians. Likewise, clients who have cognitive impairment may not be able to make informed decisions.

7. 3: Even if hospital policy allows nurses to avoid caring for clients undergoing abortions, this does not excuse the nurse from the ethical responsibility of attending to emergency situations, such as the possibility that the client is hemorrhaging. The nurse should immediately evaluate the client to determine whether emergency intervention is needed. If so, the nurse should follow protocol; if not, the nurse should reassure the client and notify the client's nurse when he or she returns.

8. 2, 4, 5, 6: These signs and symptoms are consistent with severe digoxin toxicity. The nurse should anticipate administering digoxin immune fab to counteract the digoxin. The client should have laboratory tests for digoxin and electrolyte levels (hypokalemia is common) and continuous cardiac monitoring. Supportive treatment should be provided for GI symptoms.

9. 3: The nurse should avoid using the dorsogluteal site in obese adults because adipose tissue may make it difficult to inject into the muscle. Generally, this site should be avoided if at all possible in all clients because of the danger of hitting the sciatic nerve. The deltoid muscle should be used only for small volumes of medication. The preferred site for intramuscular (IM) injections is the ventrogluteal site. When giving an IM injection in the vastus lateralis site, the tissue must be pinched and the muscle should be pulled away rather than the skin being held taut. This site is preferred for children younger than 18 months of age.

10. 2, 3, 4: If a client with Hodgkin's disease has severe pruritus that prevents him from sleeping and causes him considerable discomfort, the measures that may be most effective in relieving itching include taking the antihistamine diphenhydramine, taking opioid medications, and taking oatmeal baths. However, high humidity and high temperatures tend to aggravate itching, so the humidity is best kept at 30–40% and the temperature in the mid to low 60s. Soothing emollients applied to the skin may also provide some relief.

11. The correct order for emptying the Hemovac is:

1. V. Wash hands and apply gloves.
2. I. Open the plug on the port.
3. II. Open the Hemovac over the container, and tilt the port toward the container so the fluid drains into the container.
4. IV. Cleanse the plug and the port with an alcohol wipe in the dominant hand while compressing and holding the top and bottom of the Hemovac together with the other hand.
5. III. Place the plug into the port.

12. 4: The most likely reason for the spouse's reaction is premature completion of anticipatory grief. The spouse began the grieving process early, anticipating the loss and the emotions, and may be quite spent and emotionally withdrawn when this process completes. A different type of grieving will occur when the client actually dies.

13. 3: If a client in cervical traction complains of increasing pain in the jaw and ears, the chinstrap may be exerting excess pull on the chin, resulting in increased pressure on the temporomandibular joint. The nurse should gently correct the client's head position by tilting the head slightly forward to relieve the pull on the chin. If the pain occurs on only one side, then the traction may be uneven, and the client's body may need to be positioned correctly.

14. 2: The Safe Babies Apron is a one-piece apron that fits over the head and attaches on the side with Velcro closures. The apron contains three large pockets, one in the front and two on the sides, so the nurse can carry three infants at one time (up to 60 pounds total). Infants should be wrapped in blankets for warmth prior to being placed in the pockets. The apron is designed so the person's arms are free. This allows the nurse to carry supplies or even additional infants if necessary.

15. 1: These symptoms are indications of cardiac tamponade resulting from perforation of the ventricle and bleeding into the pericardial sac. This is a medical emergency, and the nurse must immediately notify the physician and prepare the client for surgery. Although nonhemorrhagic tamponade will usually respond well to pericardiocentesis, hemorrhagic tamponade requires a thoracotomy because the bleeding will continue until its cause is corrected.

16. 4: A patient with an ileostomy should be advised to drink about 2000 mL (8 to 10 glasses) of fluid daily because the high output of semi-liquid stool from the colostomy increases the risk of dehydration. Electrolyte levels should be monitored closely and electrolytes replaced as needed. Patients may need to further increase intake when stool output increases. In some cases, patients may be advised to take loperamide to decrease stool output if it remains excessive.

17. 2: The nurse should suspect that the client is developing acute graft versus host disease. The typical symptoms (rash, itch, and enteritis) most commonly occur within the first 100 days after transplantation and may progress to chronic graft-versus-host disease over time.

18. 2, 4, 6: Braxton Hicks contractions (false labor) begin at about six weeks of gestation and continue sporadically throughout pregnancy. Braxton Hicks contractions may be difficult to differentiate from true labor as the mother nears term, but they are characterized by contractions with no associated dilation of the cervix. Discomfort is usually felt in the lower abdomen rather than over the uterine fundus, and it does not radiate. Contractions may become rhythmic but do not become longer in duration or at closer intervals, and they may resolve with ambulation or pain medication.

19. 1: Acupuncture has been demonstrated to relieve chemotherapy-induced nausea and vomiting in a number of studies. Some studies also seem to indicate that ginger (usually in tea form) can reduce the intensity of nausea but not vomiting. The nurse may recommend both of these therapies. However, there is no evidence to suggest that therapeutic touch or magnetic therapy are effective in relieving nausea, and herbal therapies must be evaluated individually as some may interact negatively with the client's medications.

20. 2: There are 17 small boxes between any two R waves. There are 1,500 small boxes in 1 minute; therefore, the formula is:

$$1{,}500 \div \text{number of small boxes} = \text{heart rate}$$
$$1{,}500 \div 17 = 88.2, \text{which rounds to } 88$$

The R–R method of determining the heart rate is most accurate with regular rhythms and is less accurate with irregular rhythms. The R–R method is simple and can be completed rapidly.

21. 3: When changing a colostomy appliance, the skin about the stoma should be cleansed with warm tap water. Alcohol may be irritating to the tissue, and soap or baby wipes may leave residue on the tissue that interferes with adhesion. If any soap is used, it should be mild and without oils or perfume and should be rinsed off thoroughly with warm water. If skin paste is present, it should be removed before wetting the skin.

22. 4: The best approach is "What do you understand about your options for care?" The nurse should never suggest that treatment won't help because even those in hospice and palliative care receive treatment. However, the focus of treatment is different, so the nurse should stress that the goal of hospice and palliative care is to keep the client as comfortable as possible. Clients may feel they are being abandoned if the nurse suggests stopping all treatments.

23. 4: The most appropriate response to a client's complaint is to express empathy and gather information without placing blame or making excuses: "I'm so sorry you felt that way. Can you tell me what happened?" Allowing a client to ventilate feelings is often sufficient, but if the issue is serious, the nurse should describe the client's response to the nurse involved and then follow the same procedures in listening to the nurse in order to try to reach a resolution.

Mometrix

24. 2: Because attempting to evacuate clients from the facility is likely to increase exposure to the hazardous material, the most likely emergency response is to shelter in place. This applies to both staff and clients. Guidelines may vary according to the type of waste but can include locking doors, sealing doors and windows, and shutting off air-conditioning and forced-air systems. Many facilities have windows that do not open, but if not, windows should be closed immediately. Staff should monitor news reports because emergency personnel may not be readily available to provide information.

25. 4: Tardive dyskinesia (TD) is a chronic adverse effect associated with haloperidol and other neuroleptic drugs as well as anticholinergics and substances of abuse. Elderly clients and those with schizophrenia and other neuropsychiatric diseases have an increased risk of developing TD, so these drugs should be used with care or avoided. Once symptoms develop, up to 50% of clients remain afflicted, even if the medication is discontinued. No established treatment is available, although different approaches can be tried, including herbal medicines.

26. 4: If a client is experiencing hypothermia, treatment depends on the core body temperature. For a core body temperature of 28–32.2°C, active internal rewarming procedures are carried out. These include cardiopulmonary bypass, warm IV fluid administration, and warm peritoneal lavage. However, for a core body temperature of 32.2–35°C, passive or active external rewarming procedures are used. These include over-the-bed heaters and forced-air warming blankets. Patients with hypothermia have reduced sensation, so they must be carefully monitored to prevent burns.

27. 4: In this case, the initial intervention should be to call for additional help in case the situation turns violent. Then, the nurse can use techniques to try to deal with the aggression, including talking down, giving medication, removing self and others from the immediate area, and using restraints.

28. 2, 3, 4, 6: Clients with gastrointestinal disorders and diarrhea should be maintained on both standard precautions and contact precautions. The nurse should use personal protective equipment (gown and gloves) for all contact with the client but does not need to wear a mask or N95 respirator. The client should be in a private room or ≥3 feet away from other clients. Because *C. difficile* spreads readily, special care must be taken with environmental cleaning. Nurses should wash their hands with soap and water rather than alcohol antiseptic and should avoid sharing electronic thermometers used by the client with others.

29. 3: If a client is to begin hemodialysis, the best option for access is an AV fistula, which is formed by connecting an artery to a vein, usually in the lower arm above the wrist or in the upper arm. The AV fistula requires 2–3 months to mature and strengthen before it can be used for hemodialysis, so a client may have a temporary venous catheter placed during this time. An AV graft, which involves connecting an artery and vein with a synthetic vessel, matures within 2–3 weeks but is more likely to develop clotting or an infection than an AV fistula.

30. 2, 3, 4, 5: The purpose of personal protective equipment (PPE) is to protect the wearer against hazards in the workplace, so the equipment may vary from one workplace to another. Goggles, respirators, masks, gloves, and gowns are commonly used PPE in nursing, but personal radiation dosimeters may also be considered as PPE if the nurse is exposed to radiation in the workplace and needs to monitor the exposure. Back belts have not been shown in studies to reduce the risk of back injuries, are not considered PPE, and are not recommended for use.

31. 64: Pulse pressure is defined as the difference between systolic and diastolic blood pressure. In this case: 156 − 92 = 64. The normal range for pulse pressure is 30–40. A narrow pulse pressure

141

Copyright © Mometrix Media. You have been licensed one copy of this document for personal use only. Any other reproduction or redistribution is strictly prohibited. All rights reserved. This content is provided for test preparation purposes only and does not imply an endorsement by Mometrix of any particular political, scientific, or religious point of view.

(<25% of systolic reading) indicates decreased left ventricular stroke volume and can also indicate decreased cardiac output, heart failure, or shock. A widened pulse pressure may indicate a number of different conditions, including atherosclerosis, arteriovenous fistula, thyrotoxicosis, heart block, endocarditis, and pregnancy.

32. 2: Unless the client is in danger, the nurse should not confront the nurse he suspects of taking an opioid medication intended for a client because a confrontation may end badly. The other nurse may deny the accusation, place blame on the first nurse, or even react violently. Instead, the observing nurse should immediately notify a supervisor of his concerns so that the administration can carry out an investigation according to facility protocol, which also determines whether an incident report needs to be completed.

33. 1: Multifocal/multiform atrial tachycardia is a type of supraventricular tachycardia (SVT) originating from different areas within the atria, resulting in various P wave morphologies; the P wave is present but inconsistent in shape. The heart rate is usually greater than 100 bpm, and the PP intervals, PR intervals, and RR intervals are irregular. The QRS complex tends to be narrow unless there is also a bundle branch block or other abnormality. The most common cause of this condition is a pulmonary disorder such as chronic obstructive pulmonary disease, pulmonary embolism, pneumonia, hypoxia, or hypercapnia.

34. 4: As Alzheimer's disease progresses, hallucinations, delusions, and "living in the past" are very common, and trying to convince clients that what they believe is not true can often result in frustration and aggressive behavior. If the hallucinations and delusions are benign and happy memories, the nurse should allow clients to believe them and not interfere. However, if they are frightening or upsetting to the clients, then the nurse should attempt to distract the clients and refocus their attention.

35. 1, 3, 4: The following ECG tracing represents premature ventricular contraction. If occurring without other abnormalities in clients who are otherwise healthy, PVCs are usually of no particular concern and are not generally treated. PVCs may result from intake of caffeine, nicotine, or alcohol. Frequent PVCs do not signify a myocardial infarction (MI), though they can signify ventricular tachycardia if there is a run of more than 3 PVCs in a row. The presence of frequent PVCs following an MI does increase the mortality risk and must be carefully monitored. PVCs may occur in conjunction with underlying supraventricular dysrhythmias.

36. 2: While some children with pinworms (*Enterobius vermicularis*) may be essentially asymptomatic, common findings include intense anal itching and vulvovaginitis in girls. Those infected often are restless at night, sleep poorly, and may complain of intermittent abdominal pain and nausea. The tape test (tape across the anus at bedtime) is the most common diagnostic procedure because the mature worms crawl through the anus to lay eggs in the perineal folds and become attached to the tape.

37. 2: Paroxysmal supraventricular tachycardia (SVT) is sudden episodes of tachycardia originating above the ventricles because of abnormal electrical conduction in the atria or AV node. It is a dysrhythmia characterized by a regular heart rate of 150–250 bpm, abnormally shaped P waves (that may be hidden in the preceding T waves), a normal PR interval, and a normal QRS complex. The electrical discharge can originate anywhere above the bifurcation of the bundle of His. Onset is usually abrupt, and termination may be followed by a brief period of asystole. Some degree of AV block is also commonly observed.

38. 1: Inappropriate affect is a negative symptom. Schizophrenia is characterized by both negative and positive symptoms:

Positive	Negative
Hallucinations (auditory, visual, olfactory, gustatory, tactile)	Affective flattening (poor eye contact, diminished expression, inappropriate affect)
Delusions (persecution, grandeur, reference, control, somatic)	Alogia [poverty of speech] (decreased fluency and content)
Disorganized thinking and speech (echolalia, word salad, incoherence, loose association)	Avolition/Apathy (inability to initiate goal-directed activities, lack of interest in work, grooming, hygiene)
Disorganized behavior (disheveled appearance, restlessness, agitation, inappropriate sexual behavior)	Anhedonia (lack of pleasure in social activities and diminished interest in intimacy)
	Social isolation

39. 1, 2, 4, 5: The client should dispose of syringes and needles in a sharps disposal container (or glass jar) immediately after use, being sure to maintain the container out of reach of children and pets. The container should be disposed of when it is about three-quarters full because if the container is too full, the risk of accidental puncture increases. While the container may be disposed of in the regular trash in some areas, other areas are more restrictive, so the client must check with the local community garbage disposal company for guidelines. Needles should never be flushed down the toilet.

40. 2: Clients taking oral contraceptives should be advised to avoid smoking because smoking increases the risk of clot formation, which can result in heart attacks or strokes. The risk is especially high after age 35, but all women who smoke should consider an alternate method of birth control. Alcohol and diet do not increase health risks with contraceptives, although alcohol may have other negative effects. There is some evidence that women taking oral contraceptives have more muscle tenderness after exercise, but there is no increased health risk.

41. 4: When a client is terminally ill and in the end stages of life, decisions about treatment options, such as providing rehydration, should be based on whether the treatment in question provides comfort and honors the client's wishes. The consequences of treatment or no treatment must be considered. In some cases, if a client does not have an advance directive and cannot express an opinion, the decision about treatment may lie with a healthcare proxy, such as a family member.

42. 1: Agonal rhythm is often the last rhythm seen before cardiac arrest as the heart struggles. It is a cardiac emergency and is characterized by an extremely slow heart rate (<20 bpm), absent P waves, and a wide QRS complex with bizarre morphology. Agonal rhythm is not a shockable rhythm and typically leads to pulseless electrical activity, so immediate intervention is essential. An agonal rhythm is typically an indication of severe cardiac hypoxia. Causes of agonal rhythm include severe hypoxia, massive trauma or loss of blood, severe electrolyte imbalance, and drug overdose (e.g., fentanyl and other opioids).

43. 4: Weight at the 5th percentile or lower is an indication of failure to thrive. The next step after a physical exam and laboratory work is generally a dietary intake history that lists all fluid and food intake, including amounts and times, for the previous 24 hours and for the next 3–5 days, so the child's caloric and nutritional intake can be estimated. While failure to thrive may be an indication of neglect or abuse, many issues must be considered, including health condition, income, health beliefs, lack of parental education, psychosocial issues, and the child's resistance to feeding.

44. 2: The Apgar test is given at one minute and five minutes after birth to determine if emergency care is needed. A total score of 7 or above is a sign of good health.

Sign	0	1	2
Appearance (skin color)	Cyanosis or pallor over entire body	Normal, except for extremities	Entire body is normal
Pulse (heart rate)	Absent	<100 bpm	>100 bpm
Grimace (reflex irritability)	Unresponsive	Grimace	Infant sneezes, coughs, and recoils
Activity (muscle tone)	Absent	Flexed extremities	Infant moves freely
Respiration (breathing rate and effort)	Absent	Bradypnea, dyspnea	Good breathing and crying

45. 4: While a gait/transfer belt may be used by a caregiver until the client is independent, a sliding board is most indicated because the client cannot stand and requires sitting transfer. Use is quite simple and sliding boards are relatively inexpensive. They are usually made of rigid plastic material with low friction so that the client can easily slide from the chair onto the toilet or another surface. Any caregiver who will be assisting should be instructed in methods to assist the client without causing injury to the caregiver or the client.

46. 0.25: To complete the calculation, first convert micrograms (mcg) to milligrams (mg), and then dived the desired dose by the available dose:

$$(50 \text{ mcg}) \left(\frac{1 \text{ mg}}{1,000 \text{ mcg}} \right) = 0.05 \text{ mg}$$

$$\frac{0.05 \text{ mg}}{0.2 \text{ mg/tablet}} = 0.25 \text{ tablets}$$

47. 3:

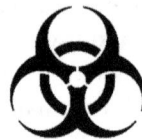

This is the international symbol for biohazards. Biohazards are biological materials, such as bacteria, viruses, and parasites, that are dangerous to people's health or pose the risk of infection. In medical facilities, items that must be labeled as biohazards include used hypodermic needles and contaminated dressings because they may contain infectious biological material. Each facility should establish protocols for handling and disposing of biohazardous materials. Biohazardous waste products are generally disposed of in red plastic bags with the biohazard symbol on the bag.

48. 1: An idioventricular rhythm occurs when the SA and AV nodes are not sending signals at a high enough rate, so the ventricle's myocardium serves as the pacemaker. The rhythm is regular, but because the intrinsic rate of the ventricles is only 20–40 bpm, the heart rate is slow. The P wave and the PR interval are absent, and the QRS complex is typically wide (>0.10 s) and may be bizarrely shaped.

49. 1: Providing basic care but refusing to talk to the client is a violation of Provision 1 of the ANA Code of Ethics for Nurses. This provision requires that the nurse practice with compassion and show respect for each individual, regardless of social/economic status, personal attributes, or type of health problems. It's the nurse's responsibility to provide care to the highest standard to all patients. Attempting to avoid caring for a particular client does not violate the Code of Ethics, but it may be construed as unprofessional.

50. 1: Indications of graft rejection in intestine recipients are often nonspecific, but an early sign may be a change in stool output. There are no specific laboratory findings that indicate rejection. Patients may develop a fever, abdominal cramping and pain, and vomiting, and the stoma may change in appearance. As rejection progresses, peristalsis may be diminished or absent, and erythema or duskiness of the graft may occur. With severe rejection, peristalsis is absent and the mucosa begins to ulcerate and slough.

51. The correct order for the states of consciousness is:

Consciousness
Wakefulness
(1) III. Arousal
Drowsiness
(2) I. Confusion
Inattentiveness
(3) II. Delirium
(4) V. Stupor
(5) IV. Vegetative state
Coma

52. 2: According to OSHA guidelines, if items are out of reach, the acceptable work practice is to get a properly maintained ladder and use that to climb up to reach the objects. The nurse should never use stools, chairs, or boxes in place of a ladder or try to "climb" up a cabinet by standing on a lower shelf. It's important to climb high enough on the ladder that the nurse is not lifting items over the head because this can result in injuries and falls.

53. 1, 3, 4: Rear-facing car seats are safest, and neonates should always be placed in rear-facing seats. Car seats should be secured in the middle of the back seat, away from airbags, or airbags should be disconnected. Neonates are at risk for hypoxia in car seats, so the parents should ensure the child's neck is straight, avoiding the chin-to-chest position, and should limit time in the car seat to short trips no longer than 60 minutes. Harnesses should be secure so that only one finger can easily slide underneath. No car seat involved in an accident should be used again even if no damage is evident.

54. 1, 2, 3: Disulfiram is a drug that alters the metabolism of alcohol, causing the level of acetaldehyde to increase markedly. This causes flushing, headache, and vertigo within minutes. The client's blood pressure falls, and he may experience syncope. He begins to vomit copiously and may experience difficulty breathing, chest pain, blurred vision, and confusion. The symptoms may persist for at least 30 minutes up to several hours, leaving the client exhausted and weak.

55. 2: An impaired nurse should not under any circumstances be allowed to care for clients, nor should Nurse A attempt to cover for the impaired nurse by observing her or assisting her with client care. Nurse A should immediately notify a supervisor of the concerns about Nurse B. Confronting another nurse about substance abuse could result in denials or even a violent confrontation, so Nurse A should not attempt to handle the situation independently.

Mometrix

56. 1, 2, 3: Difficulty urinating is a common problem after surgery, and conservative methods should be tried before catheterization. Methods to promote urination include pouring warm water over the client's perineum, asking the client to blow bubbles through a straw into a glass of water, and turning on running water while the client attempts to urinate. Telling a client to "just relax" may increase stress. It's more helpful to lead the client through relaxation exercises.

57. 4: The glucose is high normal, but both kidney function tests, the BUN and serum creatinine, are markedly elevated. This indicates a probable kidney failure, so further testing for kidney disease is indicated.

Test	Result	Normal value
BUN	172 mg/dL	7-17 mg/dL
Serum creatinine	16.4 mg/dL	8.4-10.2 mg/dL
Glucose	98 mg/dL	70-99 mg/dL

58. 2: After insertion of a Foley catheter into a male client, his penis should be positioned upward so that the catheter does not catch on his legs. It should be secured by tape to the right or left lower abdomen, with the tubing looped so the client has slack to turn from side to side. Then, the tube is taped to the edge of the bed. The tubing should hang vertically down from the mattress to the collection bag so the urine drains properly.

59. 1: When assessing a client's health history regarding intake of alcohol, the male client who goes out with friends 1 or 2 times a week and has 4–6 drinks each time would qualify as a person who is an "at-risk" drinker because he routinely drinks 4 or more drinks per occasion even though he is within the acceptable drinking range of up to 14 drinks (2 daily) per week. Females, because of differences in size and metabolism, should restrict drinking to no more than 1 drink per day.

60. 2: When assessing the fetal heart rate with the nonstress test (NST), a normal finding is at least 2 accelerations of at least 15 bpm over 15 seconds for a fetus 32 weeks or older. The normal rate is 10 bpm over 10 seconds before 32 weeks. A healthy fetus should exhibit an increased fetal heart rate with movement, and lack of accelerations may indicate hypoxemia or acidosis. However, if a 20-minute period does not show accelerations, the fetus may be in a sleeping cycle, so the testing should be extended to a 40-minute period.

61. 1, 2, 5, 6: To control exposure to dust mites, the nurse should advise the parents to keep the house clean and free of obvious dust and clutter, vacuuming frequently. They should encase the child's mattress and box spring in allergen-proof covers and wash the bed linens, pillows, clothing, and stuffed toys in hot water (>130 °F) weekly. Humidity should be maintained below 50% with a dehumidifier. It is not essential that all carpets and upholstered furniture in the home be removed, but removing these from the child's bedroom will help to decrease exposure.

62. 2: If the neonate swallowed amniotic fluid, the child may be born in acute respiratory distress, but symptoms may be delayed for a few hours, so the child must be monitored carefully. If the neonate cries at delivery and shows no signs of distress, then the mouth and throat are suctioned. If respiratory distress is evident, the child should be intubated and have tracheobronchial suctioning done to remove meconium plugs. The gastric contents may be suctioned as well to prevent the infant from regurgitating and aspirating meconium.

63. 1, 2, 3, 6: Age changes that typically occur in the respiratory system include blunting of the cough and laryngeal reflexes, making it harder to clear the lung to expel debris. Alveoli decrease in number but increase in size, making them less efficient at oxygen exchange. Ciliary action

146

decreases, increasing the risk of pneumonia. The lungs lose elasticity, and the thoracic muscles increase in rigidity. Overall, the lungs become smaller in size and have less ability to expand or expel debris. Residual volume tends to increase, so vital capacity decreases.

64. 2: To find the dosage, the first step is to convert micrograms (mcg) into milligrams (mg):

$$(112 \text{ mcg/tablet})\left(\frac{1 \text{ mg}}{1,000 \text{ mcg}}\right) = 0.112 \text{ mg/tablet}$$

Then, this value is divided into the prescribed dose:

$$\frac{0.224 \text{ mg}}{0.112 \text{ mg/tablet}} = 2 \text{ tablets}$$

65. 3: If a client is to receive two oral medications (capsules) per the enteral feeding tube, the nurse should open the capsules separately and dilute each with water. They should be drawn up in separate syringes for instilling. If the client has continuous feeding, the feeding should be stopped and the tube flushed with about 15 mL of water before instilling the first drug and then flushed again with the same volume after instillation to empty the tube of the medication before the second drug instillation. Then, the tube is flushed again before restarting the feeding.

66. 1: While protocols regarding tube feedings may vary somewhat, generally if gastric residual is less than 100 mL, it is returned to the stomach and the tubing flushed with 30 mL of water. If it is more than 100mL (in this case 150 mL), it may indicate that an obstruction has occurred, and the nurse should hold the feeding and notify the MD before proceeding. The amount of residual gastric contents should be aspirated and measured at least every 8 hours.

67. 3: With failure to capture, the heart does not respond with depolarization after a pacing spike. The ECG will show the pacing spike but no corresponding P wave or QRS complex, resulting in bradycardia. Causes of failure to capture include lead displacement, fibrosis at the lead tip, battery depletion, circuit malfunction, hyperkalemia, hypermagnesemia, cardiac ischemia, and myocardial infarction. Inappropriate pacemaker programming, such as an output setting that is too low or the incorrect pacing mode, may also result in failure to capture.

68. 4: Decorticate (flexion) posturing indicates damage to the diencephalon, decerebrate posturing indicates damage to the midbrain and pons, and flaccid posturing indicates damage to the medulla. Comas may be structural or metabolic-induced. Other assessments that may assist in determining cause include assessment of pupillary size and reaction (usually within normal limits with metabolic causes), oculomotor eye movements, and breathing patterns. CT or MRI is also used to identify structural lesions while laboratory testing may identify metabolic abnormalities, such as drug overdose.

69. 2, 3, 4, 5: When assessing a neonate's respiratory status, the following are indications of respiratory distress:

- Persistent respiratory rate at rest of > 60–70
- Flaring nostrils
- Sternal and/or intercostal retractions
- Grunting expirations

If any of these signs or symptoms are present, then the infant must undergo a thorough assessment to determine the underlying cause. The infant should be assessed for pallor or cyanosis and the lungs auscultated. The child is at risk of aspiration if the respiratory rate is above 60 when feeding.

70. 2.5: The dosage can be calculated by setting up a proportion and finding the needed volume:

$$\frac{50 \text{ mg}}{1 \text{ mL}} = \frac{125 \text{ mg}}{x \text{ mL}}$$
$$50x = 125$$
$$x = \frac{125}{50}$$
$$x = 2.5$$

The volume needed is 2.5 mL.

71. 3: Knots should always be free of the pulleys with any type of traction. If the knot lodges in the pulley, it may interfere with the line of pull, which should be along the bone axis, with the weights hanging freely. The tension rope should be in the groove of the pulley and should slide easily. The nurse should ensure that the client is lying centered on the bed because if the client's body is not aligned properly with the traction, then the line of pull may be altered.

72. 3: The nurse should tell the client that St. John's wort should not be taken with oral contraceptives because the herbal preparation increases the rate of absorption of some medications, such as oral contraceptives, decreasing their effectiveness. Acetaminophen, vitamin D, calcium carbonate, and multivitamins pose no problem.

73. 2: Two forms of identifiers should always be used prior to administering medication to any client, even if the nurse recognizes the client and is relatively sure of the client's identity. Asking the client's name and checking the hospital ID bracelet meet minimal requirements. In some cases, clients may be identified by asking their names and birthdates. The nurse should always double check the name on the medication as well. An ID bracelet that is not on the client but elsewhere, such as on a bedside stand, should not be used for identification.

74. 125: Because the child is to receive 25 mg for each kilogram of weight, the calculation is: $(25 \text{ mg/kg}) \times (10 \text{ kg}) = 250$ mg. Since the total dosage is to be given in two divided doses, the nurse will administer 125 mg at each dose.

75. 1, 2, 3, 5: Peritoneal dialysis is usually done with about 2 L of dialysate, so this means that at all times, the client retains about 2 L of fluid, which may result in slight abdominal distention. Most clients do 4–5 exchanges in a 24-hour period with a longer period of retention during the night. Each exchange usually takes 30–40 minutes. Because the fluid flows into the peritoneal cavity, the client is at risk of peritonitis, so the client must use sterile procedures.

76. 3: The "spooning" position, in which the female and her partner are lying on their sides with the male behind the female, allows penetration without undue strain on either the male or the female. The nurse should also encourage them to engage in sexual activities during the times of day when they have less pain. Taking a warm bath prior to sexual activity may also help to reduce muscle stiffness and discomfort. Intimacy is important at all ages, and the nurse should discuss the matter openly with older clients.

77. 3, 4, 5: The irrigating syringe should be filled with about 50 mL of irrigant, but it should be instilled slowly, using care not to occlude the ear canal with the syringe tip, as this may result in increased pressure and rupture of the eardrum. The client should be positioned lying flat or sitting with the head turned toward the affected ear to facilitate drainage and help secure the drainage basin. On those over 3 years old, the pinna is pulled up and back. The solution should drain out freely during the irrigation.

78. 2: Because nurses work closely with clients, a client often divulges confidential information, such as the fact that she has been having an affair with her husband's brother. However, the nurse must evaluate communications to determine if they are health related and can and should be reported or if they are private communications. In this case, no purpose is served by reporting the client's statement except to spread gossip, so this is a HIPAA violation of privacy.

79. 3, 5: Decimal numbers should contain a leading zero, such as with "0.5% albuterol inhalation solution." If the zero is missing, such as with ".25 mg budesonide inhalation solution," the initial period may be overlooked or read as a number one, and the statement may be misread as "25 mg" or "125 mg." Similarly, trailing zeroes should be avoided after whole numbers, "10 mg" instead of "10.0 mg." Abbreviations such as "SOB," which may be misinterpreted as a pejorative or as "short of breath" or "side of bed," should also be avoided and the words written out.

80. 30: Administration of medications through an NG tube under suction should be avoided if possible because some of the medication may be suctioned out; however, if medication is ordered, the nurse must disconnect the suction prior to administration, ensure the NG tube is properly placed (injecting air and listening for gurgling, aspirating, and checking the pH), flush the NG tube with 30 mL water, administer the medication, flush the tubing with another 30 mL water, and leave it disconnected from the suction for 30 minutes to allow time for the medication to be absorbed.

81. The patients should be seen in the following order:

1. I. A 6-hour postoperative client is asking for pain medication for pain of 8 on a scale of 1–10.
2. IV. A 3-day postoperative client needs assessment for sudden elevated temperature.
3. III. A 5-day postoperative client needs intermittent tube feeding.
4. II. A 2-day postoperative client needs routine dressing change.

Acute needs are handled first (pain medication and evaluation). Because a routine dressing change is not time sensitive and tube feedings are given on a regular schedule (usually every four to six hours), the tube feeding should be done before the dressing change.

82. 1, 2, 3, 5: Clients who have undergone gastric bypass surgery should avoid concentrated sugars as they accelerate emptying of the stomach. Clients should drink liquids at least 30 minutes before meals rather than with foods and should eat 5 or 6 small meals a day rather than 3 large meals. Dairy products should be restricted to low-fat products, but many people find dairy products cause diarrhea, so they should be introduced cautiously. Those with dumping syndrome may find that reclining after eating slows emptying of the stomach and reduces symptoms.

83. 3: The normal fetal heart rate (FHR) at term is 120–160 bpm; rates below this range are considered bradycardia, and rates above this range are considered tachycardia. The FHR at 5 weeks is usually around 80 bpm, increasing each day by about 3 bpm over the next month. By week 9 of gestation, the FHR has typically increased to about 175 bpm. Throughout the second trimester, the FHR is generally 120–180 bpm. However, the FHR tends to slow somewhat during the last 10 weeks before delivery.

84. 3: The nurse should realize that this is part of a death ritual and assist them in dressing the client as much as possible while treatment is still ongoing. Some cultures believe that people's souls go to the afterlife in the same clothing they wore at death, so the clothing the client is wearing at death may be very important to them.

85. 3: Intramuscular (IM) injections are almost always given to adults with a needle that is 1.0–1.5 inches in length. A shorter length (<1 inch) should be reserved for children or for very thin adults. The needle gauge usually varies from 21–25, although very thick preparations may require a gauge of 18 or 19. IM injections are usually given with a 3-mL syringe, although the maximum amount of medication in each injection should not exceed 2 mL. If larger volumes are ordered, then the dose should be divided and administered in two injections.

86. 2: The best response to the client who believes she does not need RhoGAM with a first pregnancy is the one that provides a reason why the treatment is needed: "You need treatment during your first pregnancy to prevent Rh incompatibility reactions during a second pregnancy." The serum RhoGAM contains Rh+ antibodies that agglutinate any stray fetal red blood cells that enter the mother's bloodstream to prevent antibodies forming against them because these antibodies can attack a future fetus. The mother receives RhoGAM at 26–28 weeks and again within 72 hours of delivery.

87. 3: A common psychosocial response of a pregnant client to pregnancy during the first trimester is ambivalence. Because many pregnancies are unplanned, the client may not feel prepared for motherhood or may feel apprehensive about the physical changes. Multiparas may be concerned about coping with additional children and the expenses involved in raising children. During this first trimester, pregnant women tend to be more concerned about the self than the fetus, especially if they experience morning sickness and/or mood swings associated with hormonal changes.

88. 4: A durable power of attorney for healthcare remains in effect (durable) if the client is unable to make decisions, so this is the best option. While state laws vary somewhat, a durable power of attorney for healthcare is generally limited to healthcare decisions only. In some states, a healthcare proxy can be established as part of an advance directive, but in other states two different documents are required, so the nurse should always be familiar with state regulations.

89. 1: The changes most likely represent sinus bradycardia resulting from increasing intracranial pressure. As the pulse rate falls, blood pressure increases and breathing may become irregular. Sinus bradycardia can also result from hypovolemia, although blood loss should be minimal with a fractured clavicle.

90. 1, 4, 5: If a client falls to the floor with a seizure, the nurse should avoid restraining the client or trying to insert a padded tongue blade between the teeth because this may increase injuries. However, the nurse should try to position the client on one side with the head flexed slightly forward and should support the head with cushioning of some sort to prevent head injury. Constrictive clothing should be loosened. As much as possible, the client should be provided privacy.

91. 3: This client may receive palliative care at any time since they have a life-threatening disease. While hospice care is indicated for clients whose life expectancy is 6 months or less and who are receiving no active treatment, these limitations do not apply to palliative care, which aims to provide comfort measures, such as pain control, and to allow the client to deal with the ongoing stress and needs of severe illness.

92. 4: In failure to pace, the pacemaker spikes on the ECG tracing are absent when the heart rate is slow, and there is no evidence of pacemaker activity. The tracing will only show the underlying rhythm and may indicate bradycardia or even asystole in severe cases. Causes of failure to pace include depletion of the battery, a broken or displaced lead preventing delivery of the impulse, internal circuit failure, electromagnetic interference (e.g., MRI, electrocautery, defibrillators), or incorrect programming (e.g., sensitivity settings).

93. 2: While state laws vary regarding how to report and what to report, all states require mandatory reporting of suspected child abuse. Because the type and extent of injuries to the child are not consistent with a fall off of a swing and the child has evidence of multiple previous injuries, the incident must be reported to the proper authorities. In most states, the report is made to Child Protective Services, who in turn may notify the police.

94. 2: A unit of packed red blood cells must be administered to a client within 30 minutes after removal from the blood bank refrigerator. The unit should be examined and returned to the blood bank if gas bubbles or cloudiness are evident as these may be indications of bacterial growth or hemolysis. The cells should be administered slowly (≤ 5 mL/min) for the first 15 minutes, but the flow rate can be increased after that time if the patient has no untoward reaction or is not at risk of circulatory overload.

95. 4: If an infant is to receive 65 mg of acetaminophen elixir that contains 80 mg per 5 mL, the following formula applies:

$$\frac{\text{desired dose}}{\text{available concentration}} = \text{dose volume}$$

$$\frac{65 \text{ mg}}{\frac{80 \text{ mg}}{5 \text{ mL}}} = 65 \text{ mg} \times \frac{5 \text{ mL}}{80 \text{ mg}} = \frac{65}{16} \text{mL} \approx 4 \text{ mL}$$

96. 2, 4: Latex condoms should be used one time only for each act of oral, vaginal, or anal sex and should be used only with water-based lubricants because oil-based lubricants may cause deterioration of the latex. Room should be left at the tip of the condom for sperm to collect. Latex condoms should not be used with nonoxynol-9 because this increases the risk of transmission of HIV and STDs. Condoms should be removed immediately after ejaculation before the penis becomes flaccid. No contraceptive device provides 100% protection against pregnancy, HIV, and STDs.

97. 3: The nurse should anticipate that the dosage of warfarin will be held or reduced until the INR decreases. The INR level should be maintained at 2.0–3.0 for venous thrombosis, pulmonary embolism, and valvular heart disease, and at 2.5–3.5 for clients with mechanical heart valves or recurrent systemic emboli. Vitamin K is generally not indicated as a reversal agent with an INR below 5.0, especially with no evidence of bleeding.

98. 1, 2, 5: If a client receiving treatment for breast cancer feels severely anxious, the interventions that are likely to be most effective are to instruct the client in relaxation exercises, such as deep breathing, meditation, or imagery. The nurse should encourage the client to express concerns and take the time to listen to the client as well as attempt to determine what relieves the client's anxiety and what exacerbates it in order to help the client find effective coping mechanisms.

99. 4: The metabolic effect that is most common if a client is taking a loop diuretic is hypokalemia. Therefore, clients are often prescribed supplementary potassium to take with the loop diuretic and have regular monitoring of electrolytes. Other metabolic effects that may occur are hyperglycemia and hyperuricemia. Some people may develop gastrointestinal problems, such as nausea, vomiting, and diarrhea. Other adverse effects include thrombocytopenia, neutropenia, agranulocytosis, headache, tinnitus, dizziness, and blurred vision.

100. 2: The first indication of an amniotic fluid embolism (also called pregnancy-related anaphylactoid syndrome) is usually the sudden onset of acute dyspnea because the amniotic fluid containing fetal debris (meconium, hair, skin cells, vernix) enters the maternal circulation and obstructs the pulmonary vessels, leading to acute respiratory distress followed by circulatory collapse. Because the amniotic fluid is high in thromboplastin, which interferes with clotting, the patient may develop disseminated intravascular coagulation. Maternal mortality rate is about 80%, and those who survive often have neurological impairment.

Practice Test #4

Case Study 1

The client is a 55-year-old female with a recent diagnosis of breast cancer. She had her first chemotherapy infusion 2 days ago and is being seen by her oncology team for her first follow-up visit. The client's husband has accompanied her to this appointment.

<u>NURSES' NOTES</u>

0900: Upon the nurse entering the room, the client appears weak and lethargic. She is sitting in a wheelchair clutching a trash can and groaning. When questioned about her symptoms, the client mumbles and offers incoherent answers. The client's lips are dry and cracked, and her eyes are sunken. The client's husband reports that she has had significant nausea, vomiting, and loose stools. Furthermore, the client's condition has worsened over the past 24 hours. She has been unable to eat or drink, yet continued to vomit and had diarrhea for the past 2 days.

<u>VITAL SIGNS</u>

	0900
Temp	98.9 °F axillary
HR	122, thready pulse
BP	109/70
RR	20
Pulse oximetry	98% on room air

1. Which of the following assessment findings require immediate attention? (Select all that apply.)

    1. Respiration rate
    2. Heart rate and pulse
    3. Sunken eyes
    4. Temperature
    5. Lethargy
    6. Report of continued vomiting/diarrhea

2. Based on the assessment and history for this client, the nurse anticipates that the client is most likely experiencing _____.

    1. dehydration
    2. gastroenteritis
    3. pneumonia
    4. appendicitis

3. The nurse knows to pay close attention to indications that the client's condition is worsening. The findings of _____ and _____ support the indications of worsening of the client's presenting problem. (Select 2 answers.)

    1. orthostatic hypotension
    2. crackles in the bases of the lungs per auscultation
    3. bounding pedal pulses
    4. decreased skin turgor
    5. +2 edema to the bilateral upper extremities

4. For the following list of potential interventions, specify whether each one is indicated or not indicated for the care of the client.

Potential Interventions	Indicated	Not Indicated
Closely monitor the client over the next 2 hours, and report any changes to the physician.	O	O
Initiate a D5W continuous infusion.	O	O
Encourage the client to eat a full meal.	O	O
Administer IV ondansetron.	O	O
Prepare to transfer the client to the ED for further evaluation.	O	O

NURSES' NOTES

1200: After completing treatment with IV fluids and antiemetics, the nurse reevaluates the client. The client is alert and oriented, and her skin is pink and warm to the touch. She continues to complain of nausea and has had two episodes of diarrhea.

VITAL SIGNS

	0900	1200
Temp	98.9 °F axillary	98.8 °F axillary
HR	122, thready pulse	126, thready pulse
BP	109/70	90/60
RR	20	22
Pulse oximetry	98% on room air	98% on room air

5. For the following list of assessment findings, specify whether each one indicates that the client's condition has improved, is unchanged, or has worsened.

Assessment Findings	Improved	Unchanged	Worsened
Client is alert and oriented.	O	O	O
Skin is pink and warm to the touch.	O	O	O
Client complains of nausea and diarrhea.	O	O	O
HR, 126	O	O	O
RR, 22	O	O	O
BP, 90/60	O	O	O

6. After reviewing the most recent assessment findings with the treating oncologist, the nurse anticipates new orders. Highlight all orders from the following list that the nurse should consider a priority.

- Offer the client clear liquids.
- Administer a second liter of D5W.
- Administer digoxin.
- Administer IV metoclopramide.
- Continue to monitor the client.
- Prepare the client for transport to the ED.

Case Study 2

A 68-year-old female client is brought into the emergency department via ambulance.

NURSES' NOTES

2100: A 68-year-old female arrives to the emergency department via ambulance. Emergency medical services (EMS) reports that at 2030 the client was getting ready for bed when her spouse noticed that her face was drooping and her words were no longer making sense. The client presents with a right-sided facial droop, her gaze is deviated to the left, and she does not respond when asked questions. When asked to make a fist with her right hand, the client makes a fist with her left. The client is able to blink her eyes when instructed. The client responds to touch on the left, but not on the right, and she is unable to move her right side. EMS reports that the client has a history of hypertension, type 2 diabetes, and atrial fibrillation. The client has been on lisinopril and apixaban, but she reportedly ran out last week and has been unable to get the prescriptions refilled. The client is placed on the cardiac monitor, an 18-gauge IV is placed in her left antecubital fossa, and her vital sign measurements are obtained. A bedside blood sugar level is obtained and found to be 125 mg/dL.

VITAL SIGNS

	2100
Temp	97.5 °F temporal
HR	86
BP	195/90
RR	20
Pulse oximetry	92% on room air

PHYSICAL ASSESSMENT

Body System	2100
Neurological	The client is unable to speak. She has right-sided facial droop, left gaze deviation, and no sensation or movement on the right side of her body.
Pulmonary	Lung sounds are clear; respirations are regular and unlabored.
Cardiovascular	The client is in atrial fibrillation at an irregular rate of 85–90 bpm. Heart sounds are strong; pulses are regular. No signs of chest pain. No edema noted to the extremities.

1. From the following list, select the assessment findings that require immediate follow-up. (Select all that apply.)

1. Temperature
2. Cardiovascular assessment findings
3. Neurological assessment findings
4. Blood pressure
5. Blood sugar
6. Medical history

2. For the list of client findings below, specify for each whether it is consistent with the disease processes of seizures, strokes, or hypoglycemia. Select all supported disease processes for each finding.

Client Findings	Seizure	Stroke	Hypoglycemia
Aphasia	☐	☐	☐
Gaze deviation	☐	☐	☐
Unilateral loss of sensation	☐	☐	☐
Inability to follow commands	☐	☐	☐
Facial droop	☐	☐	☐

3. Based on the clinical picture, the client is most likely experiencing a(n) _____.

1. ischemic stroke secondary to an embolism
2. ischemic stroke secondary to diabetes
3. hemorrhagic stroke secondary to a missed dose of apixaban
4. hemorrhagic stroke secondary to a fall

4. The nurse receives the following orders. Highlight all orders from the following list that the nurse should consider a priority. (Select all that apply.)

- Obtain serum blood sugar.
- Collect blood for a complete blood count (CBC), basic metabolic panel (BMP), and troponin level.
- Obtain an EKG.
- Provide education on medication compliance.
- Obtain a CT scan of the head.
- Administer IV labetalol.

NURSES' NOTES

2110: IV labetalol is administered on the way to the CT scan per the physician's orders. The client is taken to CT with the nurse and the on-call neurologist present.

2130: Upon viewing the CT scan, the neurologist confirms that there is no head bleed present, suspects that an ischemic stroke is the cause of the client's symptoms, and orders administration of a thrombolytic. Because the client is currently unable to speak, the neurologist obtains consent over the phone with the client's family. The neurologist calculates the client's initial National Institutes of Health Stroke Scale (NIHSS) score to be 24.

2135: The nurse administers the ordered thrombolytic.

VITAL SIGNS

	2100	2130
Temp	97.5 °F temporal	98.5 °F temporal
HR	86	90
BP	195/90	165/90
RR	20	18
Pulse oximetry	92% on room air	94% on room air

5. For the following list of potential nursing interventions, specify whether each is indicated or not indicated.

Potential Nursing Interventions	Indicated	Not Indicated
Regularly reassess the client's neurological symptoms.	O	O
Request an order for oral lisinopril.	O	O
Regularly recheck the client's vital signs.	O	O
Monitor for signs of facial swelling.	O	O
Request an order for physical therapy.	O	O

NURSES' NOTES

2230: The client is now able to answer orientation questions, but her speech is slurred. She still has a facial droop. The client is also now able to feel on her right side, but she states that the sensation is weaker than her left side. She is still unable to move her right side. Her gaze is still to the left, but she is now able to look to the right when directed. The nurse calculates the client's new NIHSS score to be 14.

VITAL SIGNS

	2100	2130	2230
Temp	97.5 °F temporal	98.5 °F temporal	97.4 °F temporal
HR	86	90	75
BP	195/90	165/76	190/85
RR	20	18	22
Pulse oximetry	92% on room air	93% on room air	92% on room air

6. For the following list of assessment findings, specify whether each one indicates that the client's condition has improved, is unchanged, or has worsened.

Assessment Findings	Improved	Unchanged	Worsened
Blood pressure, 190/85	O	O	O
Pulse oximetry reading, 92%	O	O	O
NIHSS score, 14	O	O	O
Facial droop	O	O	O
Gaze deviation	O	O	O

Case Study 3

An 18-month-old male client is brought in to the emergency department (ED) by his mother.

NURSES' NOTES

1600: An 18-month-old male client was rushed into the ED by his mother. His mother reports that at about 1530, the client was playing with his toys on the carpet when he suddenly fell silent, lost consciousness, and started shaking. His mother reports that his lips turned blue before he woke up. The client is now drowsy, but he will open his eyes and make brief eye contact when spoken to. The mother reports that the client has recently had a cough, has felt hot to the touch, has had a decreased appetite since the day before, and this morning had vomited up his breakfast. The client's clothes are removed, and no signs of trauma are noted. Diarrhea is found in the client's diaper. The client's weight is estimated using a Broselow tape as approximately 11 kg. The client is placed on the pediatric cardiac monitor, and a first set of vital sign measurements is obtained.

VITAL SIGNS

	1600
Temp	104 °F rectal
HR	105
BP	92/46
RR	25
Pulse oximetry	95% on room air

PHYSICAL ASSESSMENT

Body System	1600
Neurological	The client is somnolent, but he reacts to voice; eye tracking is evident.
Pulmonary	Lungs sounds are clear bilaterally. Breathing appears unlabored. Green drainage is coming from the nares, but the airway is patent.
Cardiovascular	Heartbeat is regular; pulses are strong and equal.
Integumentary	Skin is hot to the touch; cheeks are flushed. Mucous membranes are pink and moist.
Gastrointestinal	Bowel sounds are present and active. Diarrhea is found in the diaper.

1. From the following list, select the assessment findings that require immediate follow-up. (Select all that apply.)

1. Heart rate
2. Blood pressure
3. Temperature
4. Gastrointestinal assessment findings
5. Pulmonary assessment findings
6. Neurological assessment findings
7. Respiratory rate

2. For the list of client findings below, specify for each whether it is consistent with the disease processes of influenza, a urinary tract infection (UTI), or gastroenteritis. Select all supported disease processes for each finding.

Client Findings	Influenza	UTI	Gastroenteritis
Fever	☐	☐	☐
Cough	☐	☐	☐
Diarrhea	☐	☐	☐
Loss of appetite	☐	☐	☐
Rhinorrhea	☐	☐	☐

3. Based on the nurse's assessment findings, the nurse should recognize that the client most likely experienced which of the following?

1. Febrile seizure
2. Allergic reaction
3. Asthma exacerbation
4. Epileptic event

4. The nurse receives the following orders. Highlight all orders from the following list that the nurse should consider a priority.

- Obtain a urinalysis.
- Administer oral acetaminophen suspension.
- Administer oral ondansetron.
- Obtain a stool sample.
- Encourage fluids as tolerated.

5. For the following list of potential nursing interventions, specify whether each is indicated or not indicated.

Potential Nursing Interventions	Indicated	Not Indicated
Add safety padding to the sides of the client's bed.	○	○
Request that the acetaminophen order be changed to a rectal suppository.	○	○
Request an order for a 1,000 mL IV fluid bolus.	○	○
Provide the client with juice or a Popsicle.	○	○
Provide the client with a cold compress for his forehead/neck.	○	○

NURSES' NOTES

1615: With the mother's assistance, the nurse administers oral acetaminophen suspension and oral ondansetron. The nurse provides the client with a cup of apple juice and encourages the mother to assist him in drinking it as tolerated. The nurse observes the client drinking the juice with no signs of coughing or vomiting. The nurse places a pediatric urinary collection bag on the client and instructs the mother to report if the client has a wet or soiled diaper.

1700: The client's mother reports that the client has finished his juice and has not thrown up again. The client has become fussier, crying at the sight of hospital staff, and pulling at the cardiac monitor leads. The nurse notes tears are present when the client cries. A urine sample is sent to the laboratory, and the client is found to be negative for a UTI. A new set of vital signs is obtained.

159

<u>VITAL SIGNS</u>

	1600	1700
Temperature	104 °F rectal	99.5 °F rectal
Heart rate	105	140
Blood pressure	92/46	100/60
Respiratory rate	25	33
Pulse oximetry	95% on room air	98% on room air

6. The client is being prepared for discharge. Of the following statements, which indicate that the mother of the client demonstrates a good understanding of the discharge instructions? (Select all that apply.)

1. "My child was diagnosed with epilepsy today."
2. "The most accurate location to measure my child's temperature is rectally."
3. "I will alternate between acetaminophen and ibuprofen to control my child's temperature."
4. "If my child has a seizure again, I will put something in his mouth to keep him from biting his tongue."
5. "I will monitor my child's intake of fluids and have him seen again if there is a decrease in wet diapers, or if he cries without tears."

Standalone Questions

1. The following ECG tracing is an example of:

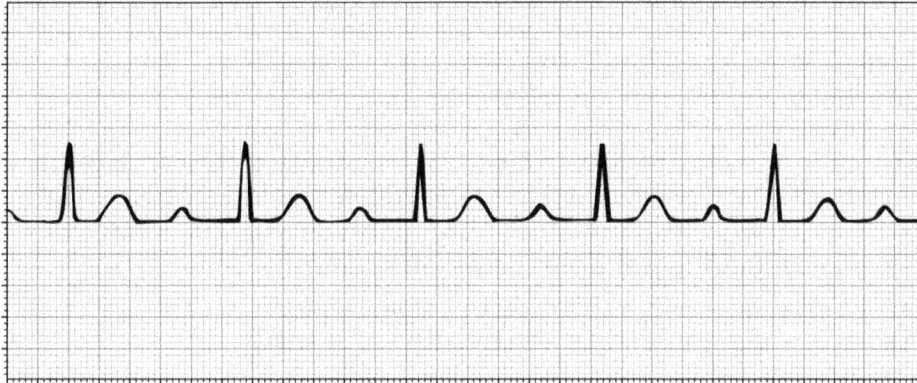

1. Sinus bradycardia
2. First-degree heart block
3. Left bundle branch block
4. Second-degree AV block

2. The nurse observes a coworker sign out a narcotic for a client. The coworker takes the medication into the nurse's restroom and returns to the nursing station without seeing the client and without the medication. Which of the following actions is most appropriate?

1. Confront the coworker about the issue.
2. Report the observation to a supervisor.
3. Report the observation the state board of nursing.
4. Monitor the coworker carefully to see if this is a pattern.

3. What physiological responses should the nurse expect when applying cold compresses to tissue? *Select all that apply.*

1. Local anesthesia
2. Increased permeability of the capillaries
3. Increased viscosity of the blood
4. Increased tissue metabolism
5. Decrease in muscle tension
6. Vasoconstriction

4. Place the following metric weight measures in the correct position in the table below.

    I. Gram
    II. Decigram
    III. Dekagram
    IV. Hectogram

Milligram	Centigram	1. ____	2. ____	3. ____	4. ____	Kilogram

161

5. A new mother is concerned that her neonate is having periods of apnea. What duration of apnea is of concern in the neonate?

1. All periods of apnea
2. 2–3 seconds
3. 6–8 seconds
4. >15–20 seconds

6. An elderly client from a long-term care facility is hospitalized for a stroke. The client has a large diamond ring that is very loose and has fallen off of their finger twice. The nurse is concerned that the ring will be lost or stolen, especially since the client has expressive aphasia. Which of the following is the best course of action?

1. Remove the ring and secure it according to hospital policy.
2. Remove the ring and send it home with the client's caregiver.
3. Leave the ring in place and tape it to the finger.
4. Leave the ring in place and take no further action.

7. Following a lumbar puncture, a client develops a severe headache that persists for 24 hours and is unrelieved by bedrest or oral fluids. Which of the following interventions does the nurse anticipate?

1. Bedrest for 3 days
2. Opioid analgesia
3. Epidural blood patch
4. Intravenous fluids

8. A client who recently tripped and fell is to begin using a rolling walker with wheels in the front only. What is the best method to properly adjust the walker to the correct height for the client?

1. Try different adjustments until one seems comfortable for the client.
2. Measure the distance from midway between the elbow and wrist and adjust the walker to that height.
3. Adjust the height so that the client can comfortably lean forward and bear weight onto the walker.
4. Measure the distance from the wrist to the floor and adjust the walker to that height.

9. A physician has ordered the HbA1c test for a client who complains of increased thirst and urination. Which of the following results (on two separate testings) is the lowest value considered diagnostic for diabetes mellitus?

1. 3.5–4.5%
2. 4.5–6.0%
3. 5.7–6.4%
4. ≥6.5%

10. A client with COPD must have the arterial blood gas (ABG) test and asks the nurse to explain the purpose of the test. Which of the following information should the nurse include? *Select all that apply.*

1. ABGs measure the levels of carbon dioxide, oxygen, and acidity in the blood.
2. ABGs help to evaluate the effectiveness of treatment.
3. ABGs measure the degree of anemia that has developed.
4. ABGs can help to determine the need for supplemental oxygen.

11. Which of the following descriptions is typical of a Parkinsonian gait?

1. Uncoordinated and unsteady, wide-based, staggering, high stepping, flat footed steps
2. Short, slow, stiff steps with thighs crossing while moving forward
3. Decreased speed and balance, slight flexion of hips and knees, stooped posture, and decreased stride length
4. Slight flexion of hips and knees, short shuffling steps, trunk leaning forward, and no arm swing

12. A client is receiving enteral feedings through a nasogastric tube, and the nurse is administering the client's medications. Which of the following can be administered through the NG tube? *Select all that apply.*

1. Hard extended-release capsules (opened, crushed, and dissolved)
2. Pills (crushed and dissolved)
3. Enteric-coated tablets (crushed and dissolved)
4. Liquid suspension
5. Soft-gel capsules (dissolved)
6. Sublingual wafer (dissolved)

13. A client in the mental health unit tells the nurse, "I drink too much because my job is so stressful and I need to relax." This is an example of which type of defense mechanism?

1. Suppression
2. Repression
3. Rationalization
4. Denial

14. The nurse must collect a urine sample for a routine urinalysis from a client who has had an indwelling Foley catheter with a sampling port for three days. After initially clamping the catheter tubing for 20 minutes, which of the following is the correct procedure?

1. The nurse collects a urine sample by inserting a needleless syringe into the sampling port and withdrawing 1 mL of urine.
2. The nurse wipes the sampling port with alcohol and then withdraws the urine using a 10-mL needleless syringe.
3. The nurse disconnects the Foley catheter from the drainage tube and allows urine to drip from the catheter into a sterile urine specimen container.
4. The nurse wipes the sampling port with alcohol, then uses a 3-ml syringe with a 1-inch 21-gauge needle to withdraw urine from the port.

15. The nurse is assisting a client to sit on the side of her bed with the bed in the low position.

> I. Support the client until she is stable.
> II. Pivot the client by moving her legs over the side of the bed and elevating her trunk.
> III. Place the client's upper arm across her chest and roll her to a side-lying position toward the nurse by pulling and supporting her shoulders and hips.
> IV. Place one arm under the client's shoulders, supporting her head and neck, and place the other arm over her thighs.
> V. Raise the head of the bed to 30° with the client in the supine position.

Place the steps (in Roman numerals) in the correct order from first to last.

> 1. _____
> 2. _____
> 3. _____
> 4. _____
> 5. _____

16. The nurse is concerned that the procedures commonly used for wound care are outdated and wants to move toward a more evidence-based approach. Which of the following is the best place to begin to gather information?

1. Survey physicians.
2. Search medical databases.
3. Look through books in the medical library.
4. Contact healthcare providers specializing in wound care.

17. A registered nurse is assigned as team leader for an LPN and two CNAs. The registered nurse must delegate a number of different tasks:

- Dressing change on a foot ulcer
- Insertion of a Foley catheter
- Enema as prep for a radiological procedure
- Bed baths for four clients
- Checking routine vital signs

Which task(s) may be delegated to the LPN by the RN?

1. Dressing change only
2. Dressing change and insertion of a Foley catheter
3. Dressing change and enema
4. Dressing change, enema, and insertion of Foley catheter

18. Using Naegele's rule for estimating the due date for a pregnancy, if a client's last menstrual cycle started on September 6 and ended September 10, when is the client's approximate due date?

1. June 6
2. June 13
3. June 10
4. June 17

19. Which of the following are examples of autoimmune disorders? *Select all that apply.*

1. Guillain-Barré syndrome
2. Diabetes mellitus, type 1
3. Rheumatoid arthritis
4. Hashimoto thyroiditis
5. Osteoarthritis
6. Diabetes mellitus, type 2

20. For which of the following reasons are benzodiazepines usually avoided in frail older adults?

1. May result in respiratory depression
2. May increase risk of falls
3. May increase risk of osteoporosis
4. May increase risk of hypertension

21. When reviewing dietary restrictions with an immunocompromised client following kidney transplantation, the client should be advised to avoid which of the following food products?

1. Raw bean sprouts
2. Strawberries
3. All citrus fruits
4. Milk products

22. A client with schizophrenia has frequent hallucinations and is becoming increasingly withdrawn. Which of the following are appropriate interventions for hallucinations? *Select all that apply.*

1. Communicate frequently with the client to help present reality.
2. Use distracting techniques.
3. Ask the client to describe the hallucinations.
4. Encourage the client to participate in reality-based activities, such as playing cards.
5. Tell the client to ignore the hallucinations.

23. A client has suffered an ischemic stroke in the right hemisphere. Which of the following should the nurse anticipate?

1. Left-sided paralysis and visual field defects
2. Expressive, receptive, and/or global aphasia
3. Uncharacteristic positive attitude and outlook
4. Difficulty with mathematics, reading, and writing

24. Which of the following foods has the greatest potential for interaction with drugs?

1. Milk products
2. Grapefruit
3. Potatoes
4. Cabbage

25. The nurse is providing education about Raynaud's disease to a 35-year-old female client. Which of the following information should the nurse include? *Select all that apply.*

1. Stop smoking (make a referral to a smoking cessation program).
2. Wear mittens and gloves when outside during cold weather.
3. Avoid calcium channel blockers.
4. Avoid vasodilators.
5. Avoid birth control pills.

26. Which of the following pulmonary changes are associated with aging? *Select all that apply.*

1. Decreased pulmonary elasticity
2. Increased alveolar surface area
3. Increased chest-wall rigidity
4. Increased forced vital capacity
5. Decreased laryngeal reflexes

27. An older client says that she frequently experiences stress incontinence and may have to stop playing golf because swinging the golf club often results in small amounts of urinary incontinence. Which of the following suggestions will likely be most effective?

1. Take a deep breath while swinging the golf club.
2. Utilize the "knack" (precisely timed muscle contractions).
3. Wear incontinence pads.
4. Urinate immediately before playing golf.

28. If a client who had abdominal surgery the previous day experiences evisceration and the nurse finds intestines protruding from the wound, what initial step should the nurse take to protect the wound?

1. Cover with saline-soaked sterile dressings.
2. Cover with a dry sterile dressing.
3. Cover the wound with plastic.
4. Leave the wound exposed to air.

29. A client who was prescribed increasing dosages of baclofen to relieve muscle spasms should have taken 80 mg daily in four divided doses but misunderstood and took 80 mg four times a day, resulting in an overdose and pronounced CNS depression. Which of the following treatments does the nurse anticipate?

1. Administration of naloxone
2. Administration of atropine
3. Supportive care only
4. Administration of flumazenil

30. Which cephalic presentation is most common during delivery of a neonate?

1. Vertex
2. Face
3. Military
4. Brow

31. A client has recorded her intake as follows:

8 oz. tea	4 oz. ice cream
4 oz. gelatin dessert	8 oz. water
6 oz. apple juice	6 oz. milk

The nurse must record the fluid intake in milliliters. How many milliliters of fluid intake will the nurse record for this client? *Record your answer as a whole number.*

_____ mL

32. During the second stage of labor, the baby's head becomes compressed because the mother has a narrow, bony pelvis. Which of the following is the most common result for the infant from this type of compression?

1. Cerebral palsy
2. Intracranial hemorrhage
3. Cranial molding
4. Epilepsy

33. A 52-year-old client is undergoing menopause. Which of the following physical signs or symptoms is often attributed to the decreased estrogen production associated with menopause?

1. Weight loss
2. Excessive sleeping
3. Increased fat deposits on hips and abdomen
4. Increased metabolic rate

34. Following a client's death, the nurse helps the client's daughter reposition the client, and the daughter insists that she heard the client breathe as the client was moved. Which of the following is the best response?

1. Tell the daughter she was mistaken about hearing respirations.
2. Listen to the client's lungs for signs of respirations to reassure the daughter.
3. Explain that trapped air escaped from the lungs when the client was moved.
4. Tell the daughter that the sound she heard was normal after death.

35. A 4-year-old child with autism spectrum disorder has verbal skills but interacts poorly. The child says "bunny" and reaches for a stuffed animal that is on a shelf. Which of the following is the best example of incidental teaching?

1. The nurse asks, "What color is the bunny?" and waits for a response before giving the child the toy.
2. The nurse states, "That's right! That is a bunny," and gives the child the toy.
3. The nurse gives the child the toy without comment.
4. The nurse states, "Before you get the bunny, you need to answer some questions."

36. What type of pacemaker malfunction is demonstrated by the following ECG tracing?

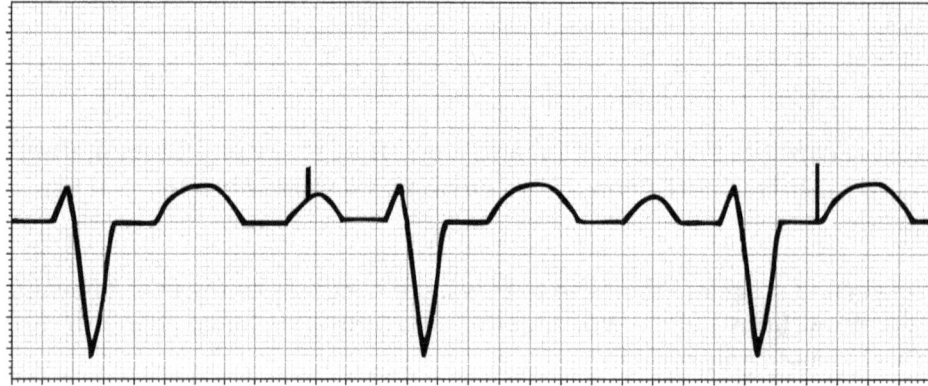

1. No malfunction
2. Failure to sense
3. Failure to capture
4. Failure to pace

37. If a client with bipolar disorder is exhibiting disturbed thought processes as evidenced by delusional thinking, which of the following is the most appropriate response?

1. "You are wrong about what you are thinking."
2. "Try to think about this logically, and you'll see what you believe is impossible."
3. "I understand you believe this, but I don't see evidence that this is true."
4. "Look around. You are the only person who believes this!"

38. A client has suffered a severe traumatic brain injury and is being treated in the ICU. Which of the following interventions does the nurse anticipate to control intracranial pressure? *Select all that apply.*

1. Elevate the head of the bed.
2. Administer oxygen to maintain a SpO2 above 90%.
3. Maintain neutral alignment of the head.
4. Administer sedation to prevent or reduce agitation.
5. Maintain body temperature below normal limits.

39. A client's medication order is for 300 mg of a liquid medication that is available at 75 mg per mL. How many mL should the nurse administer to the client? *Record your answer as a whole number.*

_____ mL

40. A 15-year-old client took a full bottle of extra-strength acetaminophen in a suicide attempt 5 hours prior to admission to the emergency department for treatment, and the serum level of the drug is 180 mcg/mL. Which of the following interventions does the nurse anticipate? *Select all that apply.*

1. Antidote: 72-hour N-acetylcysteine (NAC) protocol
2. Supportive care
3. GI decontamination with activated charcoal
4. Monitoring of hepatic function
5. Psychiatric consultation

41. The nurse is caring for a client in the recovery room after the client's abdominal surgery. The client's base BP prior to surgery was 130/84. The recovery room BP record is as follows:

- 1:00 PM 126/84
- 1:15 PM 128/82
- 1:30 PM 124/80
- 1:45 PM 116/72
- 2:00 PM 110/66
- 2:15 PM 100/62

Which of the following is the most appropriate response?

1. Notify the surgeon of the change in BP.
2. Continue to monitor the client as usual.
3. Increase the rate of oxygen flow to the client.
4. Notify the surgeon if the systolic BP falls below 90.

42. A client has acute central nervous system edema, due to spinal cord injury. The drug of choice for controlling this patient's edema is:

1. Aspirin
2. Mannitol
3. Morphine
4. Methylprednisolone

43. A client has had a central catheter inserted for administration of parenteral nutrition. An x-ray was taken to ensure correct positioning prior to commencing infusions. The x-ray report indicates that the catheter tip is in the right atrium. Which of the following actions by the nurse is correct?

1. Hold the infusion and notify the MD.
2. Gently withdraw the catheter 2–3 inches.
3. Begin the infusion as the catheter is placed correctly.
4. Gently insert the catheter 2–3 inches further.

44. The nurse is examining a client's incision following a radical nephrectomy. Which of the following signs or symptoms may be most indicative of infection? *Select all that apply.*

1. Slight serosanguineous discharge is evident on the dressing.
2. Tissue around the incision is moderately edematous and increasingly erythematous.
3. The dressing that has covered the incision has a foul odor.
4. The client has pain in the incisional area.
5. There is purulent discharge from the wound.

45. A client has accidentally splashed a toxic (although not caustic) substance in his right eye, and the nurse must flush the eye. Which of the following steps are correct? *Select all that apply.*

1. Position the client's head down until level and on the left side.
2. Irrigate with a bulb syringe tip about a half-inch above the eye.
3. Flush for about 5 minutes.
4. Hold the eyelid open with thumb and index finger while flushing.
5. Hold an emesis basin against the left side of the client's face to contain the irrigant.

46. During which stage of injury repair does the wound show evidence of erythema and edema and phagocytosis begin?

1. Proliferation
2. Inflammation
3. Hemostasis
4. Maturation

47. A client with epilepsy is taking phenytoin. What long-term effects should the nurse advise the client can occur with prolonged administration of phenytoin? *Select all that apply.*

1. Gingival hypertrophy
2. Hirsutism
3. Hypertrophy of facial subcutaneous tissue
4. Dementia
5. Anemia

48. A client recently diagnosed with colon cancer becomes furious when the nurse gives her an injection, shouting, "You hurt me, you idiot! You are so incompetent!" Which of the following is the most likely reason for the outburst?

1. The nurse is incompetent.
2. The client is in the anger stage of the grief response.
3. The client is in the denial stage of the grief response.
4. The client has a low pain tolerance.

49. Clients taking anticholinergic drugs, such as benztropine mesylate, to relieve muscle tremors and muscle rigidity associated with Parkinson disease should be advised to avoid which of the following?

1. Overheating
2. Overeating
3. Excessive fluid intake
4. Skipping meals

50. Which of the following are examples of positive reinforcement for a client with anorexia? *Select all that apply.*

1. The nurse tells the client, "If you don't stay with the program, you won't make progress."
2. The client is granted an additional hour of Internet use after eating all her dinner.
3. The nurse tells the client, "You are making good progress."
4. The client gains one-half pound.
5. The client loses privileges for losing one-half pound.

51. When inserting a nasogastric feeding tube, the nurse pauses after inserting about 25 cm of tubing, listens at the distal end of the tubing, and hears air exchange. Which of the following is the most appropriate response?

1. Continue to insert tube but withdraw if coughing becomes excessive.
2. Continue to slowly insert tube while the patient swallows sips of water.
3. Pull the tube back approximately 10 cm and then reinsert.
4. Remove the tube and start the procedure again.

52. A client is to receive 120 mL of normal saline per hour intravenously. The drop factor is 15 drops per mL. What drip rate should the nurse set in drops per minute? *Record your answer as a whole number.*

_____ drops/minute

53. A physician has telephoned a number of orders for a client who has developed a fever and chills. Which of the following is the correct procedure when taking telephone orders?

1. Write the orders directly into the client's record as given.
2. Write the orders in their entirety and then read them back and confirm.
3. Repeat each order one at a time and ask for confirmation for each before proceeding.
4. Insist the physician email or fax a copy of the orders for confirmation.

54. A client with Alzheimer's disease has repeatedly gotten out the front door at night and run away. Which of the following suggestions may be helpful to a caregiver? *Select all that apply.*

1. Hang a curtain over the front doorway.
2. Place a latch at the top or bottom of the front door.
3. Lock the client into her bedroom.
4. Place a motion sensor with a loud alarm on the client's bedroom door.
5. Place bed restraints on the client.

55. The nurse notes that a transfer procedure is time consuming because of redundant steps and has developed a streamlined procedure. The nurse should:

1. Personally use the streamlined procedure.
2. Tell the other staff members to use the streamlined procedure.
3. Propose the new procedure to the performance improvement committee.
4. Print up instructions for the new procedure and let others decide whether to use it.

56. A client that is homeless has been treated in the emergency department for a small cut received in a fight with another homeless person and is about to be discharged after suturing. Which of the following information would be most helpful for the client, in addition to information about wound care and a follow-up appointment?

1. Telephone number for Adult Protective Services
2. Telephone number of the police department
3. List of shelters and community agencies
4. List of 12-step organizations

57. Identify the abnormality seen in the ECG below.

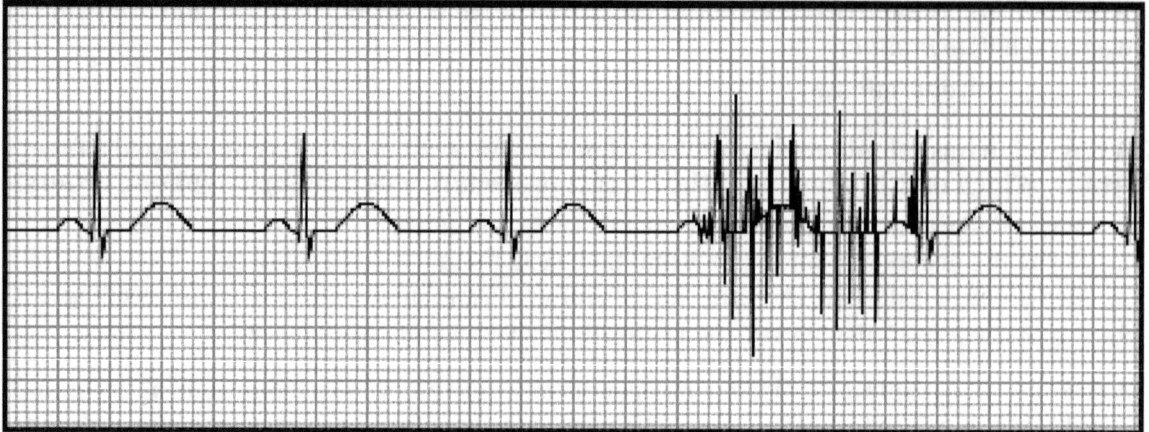

1. Atrial flutter
2. Transient supraventricular tachycardia
3. Ventricular fibrillation
4. Muscle tremor

58. A client with multiple sclerosis tires easily, so the nurse is instructing the client in energy-conservation techniques. Which of the following techniques may help the client conserve energy? *Select all that apply.*

1. Sit down to perform activities instead of standing.
2. Keep frequently used items close at hand on the floor or on a high shelf.
3. Rest 10 minutes out of every hour.
4. Plan ahead to avoid extra movements.
5. Watch for stress signals, such as dyspnea or fatigue.
6. Pull objects instead of pushing them.

59. A client has been admitted through the emergency department after an acute episode of GI hemorrhage. The client's hemoglobin is 6.1 and hematocrit is 18.3. The client is a Jehovah's Witness and has refused transfusions even though his hemoglobin and hematocrit are still falling; the physician has advised him that he might die without transfusions. Which of the following is the most appropriate response for the nurse?

1. Provide supportive care and respect the client's right to refuse treatment.
2. Urge the client to consider his family and reconsider his decision.
3. Tell the client that his decision is unreasonable.
4. Ask the client's family members to reason with the client.

60. A physician has prescribed nortriptyline hydrochloride, a tricyclic antidepressant, for a client with postherpetic syndrome who prefers not to take opioids because of a history of substance abuse. When discussing use of the drug with the client, which of the following information should the nurse include? *Select all that apply.*

1. The medication should be taken at bedtime.
2. The medication must be taken with food.
3. The client may need to take a stool softener.
4. The client should report urinary dysfunction.
5. The client may experience sexual dysfunction.

61. A client with a head injury is being admitted into the intensive care unit with a score on the Glasgow Coma Scale of 6. Based on this score, what condition does the nurse anticipate?

1. Mild head injury
2. Severe head injury
3. Coma
4. Moderate head injury

62. A client has recurrent episodes of constipation and fecal impaction. The nurse is assisting the client with a bowel-training regimen. Which of the following interventions should be included? *Select all that apply.*

1. Scheduled toileting
2. Stool softeners
3. High-fiber diet
4. Daily laxatives
5. Periodic enemas
6. Routine exercise

63. If a nurse must move a heavy cart full of supplies, which of the following techniques uses the best body mechanics?

1. Push the cart from behind with both hands, keeping the head up and back straight.
2. Pull the cart from ahead with one hand, leaning forward slightly.
3. Push the cart from behind, pushing against it with the shoulders.
4. Pull the cart from ahead with one hand, keeping the head up and back straight.

64. While the nurse is accessing a client's electronic medical record, a coworker (not assigned to the client) leans over the nurse and begins to read the client's record. The nurse should:

1. Allow the coworker to read the record.
2. Ask the coworker to stop reading.
3. Immediately block their view or close-out the screen.
4. Threaten to report the nurse to a supervisor.

65. A client receiving total parenteral nutrition (TPN) exhibits a sudden onset of respiratory distress with cough and dyspnea, and oxygen saturation level falls to 88%. On examining the client, the nurse finds that the IV tubing has become disconnected so that part of the catheter system is open to the air. The immediate response before notifying the physician should be to:

1. Clamp the catheter and place client in left lateral Trendelenburg position.
2. Clamp the catheter and place the client in supine position with the head of the bed elevated.
3. Reconnect the tubing immediately and provide oxygen.
4. Remove the catheter and provide oxygen.

66. A client is to be discharged with a tracheostomy. Which of the following should the nurse most stress when educating the client about home management? *Select all that apply.*

1. Bowel care
2. Pulmonary hygiene
3. Dietary supplements
4. Tracheostomy care
5. Exercise program

67. What does this ECG tracing illustrate?

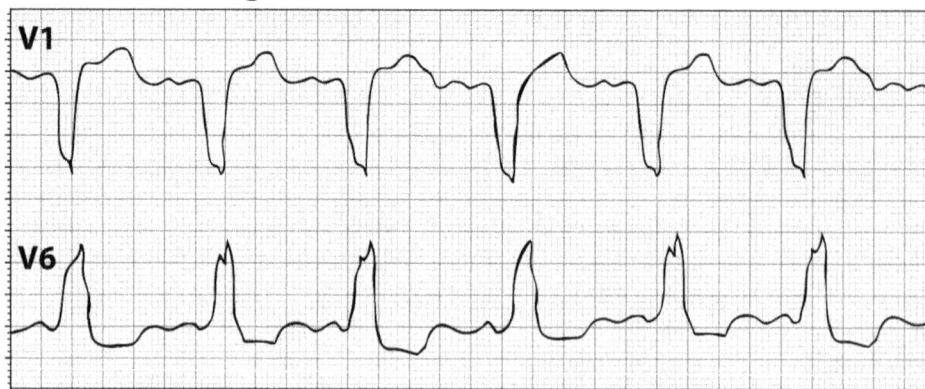

1. Normal sinus rhythm
2. Left bundle branch block
3. Right bundle branch block
4. Left ventricular hypertrophy

68. A 78-year-old client with a history of diabetes mellitus type 2, GERD, and hypertension is hospitalized with pneumonia. The client rings the call bell at 11 p.m., complaining of being unable to sleep and having "indigestion" and "heartburn." Which of the following initial interventions is most indicated?

1. Administer antacid per prn order.
2. Administer acetaminophen per prn order.
3. Administer hypnotic per prn order.
4. Assess cardiac and respiratory status.

69. If the nurse examining the blisters of a client in the active phase of herpes zoster (shingles) has direct contact with bare hands to the fluid in some of the blisters, the nurse may be at risk of developing which of the following?

1. Herpes zoster (shingles)
2. Varicella zoster virus (chickenpox)
3. Viral meningitis
4. There is no risk of transmission.

70. A nurse is concerned that current procedures for wound care are not adequate and would like to propose changes. When pursuing process improvement, where should the nurse begin?

1. Survey literature regarding wound care.
2. Conduct interviews of physicians.
3. Dispense staff questionnaires.
4. Ask permission of the director of nursing.

71. The nurse must teach a female client to carry out clean intermittent catheterization (CIC). The steps to the procedure (in Roman numerals) include:

> I. Locate meatus (by touch or with mirror).
> II. Insert catheter and hold in place until urine stops draining.
> III. Spread labia and cleanse area with soap and water.
> IV. Lubricate catheter (with water soluble lubricant).

Place the steps in Roman numerals the correct order.

> 1. _____
> 2. _____
> 3. _____
> 4. _____

72. A nulliparous client has been admitted after 12 hours of mild contractions at home. On examination, the client is found to be fully effaced and dilated to 3 cm. Contractions are every 5 minutes and last approximately 60 seconds. The client asks the nurse approximately how long it should take to get to 10 cm dilation. Which of the following is the most appropriate response?

> 1. Approximately 3 hours
> 2. Approximately 4 hours
> 3. Approximately 5 hours
> 4. Approximately 7 hours

73. The nurse is working in a hospital unit when a tornado levels a large shopping mall near the hospital, resulting in mass casualties. The hospital is on alert and has advised staff that hospital beds must be freed for incoming injured. What immediate action should the nurse take?

> 1. Wait for further directions.
> 2. Inform current clients they will probably be discharged.
> 3. Make a list of noncritical clients who might be safely discharged.
> 4. Start calling physicians to ask if their clients can be discharged.

74. A 4-year-old client weighing 39.6 pounds is to receive an infusion of IV ceftriaxone sodium at 75 mg/kg/d in a divided dose every 12 hours. How many mg should the child receive with each infusion? *Record your answer as a whole number.*

> _____ mg

75. Which of the following fractures poses the greatest risk for older adults?

> 1. Wrist
> 2. Vertebral
> 3. Radial/ulnar
> 4. Hip/femur

76. A client is admitted for treatment of a myocardial infarction but insists on leaving against medical advice (AMA). The nurse has attempted to reach the physician, who has not responded. Which of the following measures should the nurse take? *Select all that apply.*

1. Advise the client of health risks of leaving before treatment is completed.
2. Assess the client's mental status and ability to make decisions.
3. Ask the client to sign an AMA form.
4. Arrange for follow-up by phone or return visit.
5. Advise the client that he cannot leave until the physician arrives.

77. A client in the mental health unit has a panic-level anxiety attack and has become immobile, mute, and is not processing environmental stimuli. Which of the following actions is the best nursing response?

1. Attempt to distract the client through music or conversation.
2. Remain with the client and speak in a calm, reassuring voice.
3. Remind the client that the anxiety will pass.
4. Encourage the client to use self-hypnosis techniques.

78. If a client has had a repair of a right fractured hip and has an overhead trapeze on the bed to assist with movement, which of the following instructions should the client receive about use of the assistive device? *Select all that apply.*

1. The client should always grasp the bar with both hands before moving.
2. The client should grasp the bar with the left hand and place the right hand flat on the bed to assist with movement.
3. The client should flex the left hip and knee and place the foot flat on the bed before moving.
4. The client should keep the left hip and knee extended when moving.

79. A client has had four pregnancies. She experienced one miscarriage at 12 weeks, had one stillborn birth at 34 weeks, a healthy son at 38 weeks, and a healthy daughter at 40 weeks. How would the client's obstetric history be classified?

1. Gravida 3, Para 2
2. Gravida 4, Para 4
3. Gravida 4, Para 3
4. Gravida 4, Para 2

80. The nurse must give a client a nebulizer treatment every 4 hours. When is the most appropriate time to document the treatments in the electronic health record?

1. At the beginning of the nurse's shift
2. Immediately after each treatment
3. Within 2 hours of each treatment
4. At the end of the nurse's shift

81. If a long-time user of opioids is administered naloxone (Narcan) for an opioid overdose, which of the following may occur as a result of the reversal agent?

1. Parkinsonian-like tremors
2. Confusion and disorientation
3. Hyperthermia
4. Withdrawal and seizures

82. When assessing a 75-year-old client for risk of falls, the nurse conducts the timed up and go (TUG) test. What is the normal time required for a client to complete standing, walking 3 meters, turning, returning back, and sitting down?
   1. 4–6 seconds
   2. 7–10 seconds
   3. 11–14 seconds
   4. 15–20 seconds

83. The nurse is opening a sterile dressing pack to change the dressing on a client's abdominal wound. Which of the following actions will contaminate the contents of the pack?
   1. The nurse holds the sterile dressing below waist level when transferring it to the sterile drape.
   2. The nurse holds the package in his nondominant hand while peeling the wrapper over the nondominant hand with his other hand.
   3. The nurse positions the bottom half of the sterile drape over the top half of the work surface before placing the top half of the drape over the bottom half of the work surface.
   4. The nurse opens the outermost flap of the sterile kit away from his body.

84. If the nurse has made a medication error, giving the wrong client a dosage of antacid, which of the following is the appropriate action?
   1. No action is required as antacids are harmless.
   2. Notify the physician, document the medication given, and file an incident report.
   3. Notify the physician only.
   4. Ask the physician for a retroactive order for an antacid.

85. A client with heart failure has a left ventricular ejection fraction of 38%. When educating the client about managing the condition, which of the following advice should the nurse include? *Select all that apply.*
   1. The client should take frequent rest periods.
   2. The client should avoid strenuous activities.
   3. The client should stop all exercises.
   4. The client should stop smoking.
   5. The client should limit alcohol intake to 2–3 drinks daily.

86. A client has experienced repeated panic attacks and periodically snaps a rubber band against his wrist during a visit to a clinic. Which of the following is the most likely reason for this action?
   1. The client has a nervous habit.
   2. The client is practicing self-injurious behavior.
   3. The client is trying to get attention.
   4. The client is practicing thought-stopping.

87. Which of the following dressing types is most appropriate for a stage II pressure injury with moderate amounts of exudate?
   1. NS on gauze (wet-to-dry)
   2. Transparent film
   3. Hydrocolloid
   4. Hydrogel

88. The nurse is planning to empty a Jackson-Pratt drainage device for a client following a mastectomy. Before emptying the bulb, the nurse notes a number of large clots in the tubing. Which of the following is the most appropriate response?

1. Leave the clots undisturbed.
2. Notify the physician that the device needs to be changed.
3. Irrigate the tubing with normal saline.
4. Milk the tubing before emptying the device.

89. The nurse should advise a client who plans to get pregnant to take which of the following vitamins or minerals to prevent neural tube defects?

1. Vitamin D
2. Vitamin B9 (folic acid)
3. Vitamin C
4. Iron

90. Which of the following are required components of an informed consent? *Select all that apply*.

1. Duration of procedure
2. Alternative options
3. Nature and reason for procedure
4. Risks and benefits
5. Explanation of diagnosis

91. A client has been diagnosed with Parkinson's disease and has been prescribed levodopa. Which of the following are contraindications to levodopa? *Select all that apply*.

1. Narrow-angle glaucoma
2. Macular degeneration
3. Pregnancy
4. Melanoma
5. Cataracts

92. Which of the following are examples of normalization for pediatric clients? *Select all that apply*.

1. Painting children's rooms in bright colors
2. Providing a play area
3. Allowing siblings to visit
4. Facilitating doll reenactment play
5. Serving meals on trays in children's rooms

93. A client who is 2 months pregnant states that she has never received a measles vaccination and was exposed to a child with measles 14 days earlier. The client asks the nurse if she is still at risk of developing measles. Which of the following is the most accurate information?

1. The client is no longer at risk.
2. The client is at risk for another 2 days.
3. The client is at risk for another 7 days.
4. The client is at risk for another 14 days.

94. A client with a brain tumor has exhibited changes in mood and personality and has developed weakness on her right side. Based on these symptoms, the nurse suspects the tumor is located in which part of the brain?

1. Occipital lobe
2. Frontal lobe
3. Temporal lobe
4. Cerebellum

95. The nurse is to administer 250 mL of normal saline intravenously with a flow rate of 15 drops per minute and a drop factor of 15 drops/mL. How many minutes will it take to complete the infusion? *Record your answer as a whole number.*

_____ minutes

96. When assessing a client's skin, the nurse notes a scattered red rash on the trunk. The individual lesions are about 0.5 cm in diameter and are flat, nonpalpable, and circumscribed. How would this type of lesion be classified?

1. Papule
2. Nodule
3. Macule
4. Patch

97. The nurse is assessing a client's cardiac monitoring and notes the following electrocardiogram (ECG) recording:

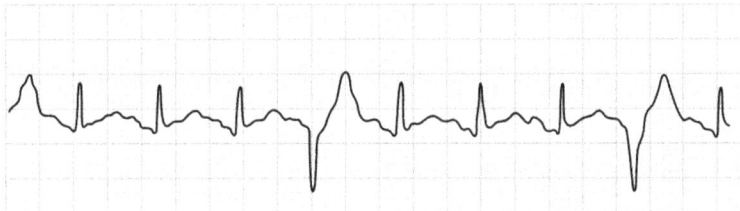

How would the nurse classify this cardiac abnormality?

1. Atrial flutter
2. Premature junctional contraction
3. Ventricular tachycardia
4. Premature ventricular contraction

98. The nurse has to apply a warm moist compress to an abscessed area on the back of a client's neck. What is the temperature range for a warm compress?

1. 37–41 °C (98–106 °F)
2. 34–37 °C (93–98 °F)
3. 26–34 °C (80–93 °F)
4. 18–26 °C (65–80 °F)

99. An 11-year-old child with autism spectrum disorder is hospitalized. Whenever his parents are not present, he gets extremely agitated, refuses to take his medications, screams, and hits his head against the bed headboard. Which of the following is likely the most effective method of controlling the child's behavior?

1. Ask the parents for advice.
2. Ask the physician for a sedative.
3. Place the child in restraints.
4. Ask a physician for a psychiatric referral.

100. The nurse has inserted a nasogastric tube and aspirated gastric contents to check the pH with color-coded pH paper. The aspirate is dark brown, and the pH measures at 5 according to the color chart. What does this pH usually indicate?

1. Gastric aspirate
2. Intestinal aspirate
3. Respiratory aspirate
4. Inconclusive results

Answer Key and Explanations for Test #4

Case Study 1

1. 2, 3, 5, 6: The client presents with altered mental status, changes to pulse, and sunken eyes, which are significant changes in condition that warrant urgent intervention. Uncontrolled vomiting and diarrhea need to be addressed to prevent further decline. The respiration rate is within normal limits. The blood pressure reading is low, but not critical. The client is afebrile.

2. 1: Given the client's presentation, coupled with the subjective report of nausea, vomiting, and diarrhea lasting 2 days and worsening over the course of the past 24 hours, the client is most likely experiencing dehydration secondary to her chemotherapy treatment. Gastroenteritis can also result in dehydration, but this is not the likely causative factor given the client's history. The client is afebrile and does not present with respiratory symptoms; therefore, pneumonia is unlikely. Although appendicitis can present with nausea and vomiting, the pain is more acute and specific to the right lower quadrant.

3. 1, 4: Orthostatic hypotension (i.e., a lowering in blood pressure from sitting to standing) and decreased skin turgor (i.e., the elasticity of the skin) are findings that indicate that the dehydration is worsening and starting to impact multiple body systems. Bounding pedal pulses, crackles in the lungs, and edema are not commonly associated with dehydration; rather, these symptoms can be associated with hypervolemia or congestive heart failure.

4.

Potential Interventions	Indicated	Not Indicated
Closely monitor the client over the next 2 hours, and report any changes to the physician.	●	○
Initiate a D5W continuous infusion.	●	○
Encourage the client to eat a full meal.	○	●
Administer IV ondansetron.	●	○
Prepare to transfer the client to the ED for further evaluation.	○	●

Given the significant changes to the client's condition over a short period of time, the physician will want to closely monitor the client and initiate symptom management measures as soon as possible. Intravenous (IV) fluids would be ordered to replace lost hydration, and antiemetics would be ordered to stop the nausea and vomiting. Oral intake would be discouraged until digestive symptoms have subsided. The client's current condition does not warrant evaluation in the ED at this point.

5.

Assessment Findings	Improved	Unchanged	Worsened
Client is alert and oriented.	●	○	○
Skin is pink and warm to the touch.	●	○	○
Client complains of nausea and diarrhea.	○	●	○
HR, 126	○	●	○
RR, 22	○	○	●
BP, 90/60	○	○	●

Finding the client alert and oriented with a normalized skin appearance indicates an improved condition. Nausea and diarrhea have not yet subsided and remain unchanged from the previous assessment. The client remains tachycardic, though the slight increase in heart rate is not a clinically significant increase. The client's respiratory rate (now representing tachypnea) and blood pressure (representing profound hypotension) have both worsened and are indicative of severe hypovolemia/dehydration.

6.

- Offer the client clear liquids.
- Administer a second liter of D5W.
- Administer digoxin.
- Administer IV metoclopramide.
- Continue to monitor the client.
- Prepare the client for transport to the ED.

The client has improved slightly, although not as much as needed, necessitating continued intervention with IV fluids and antiemetics. The client should continue to be monitored closely for any changes to her status. Given the continued gastrointestinal symptoms, a clear liquid diet would not be encouraged yet. Digoxin is not indicated because the client is not in heart failure. The client's current status does not necessitate transport to the ED.

Case Study 2

1. 3, 4, and 6: The client's temperature, cardiovascular assessment, and blood sugar are all expected findings given her medical history. The client's neurological assessment and elevated blood pressure are abnormal findings that require further testing emergently. The client's medical history shows that she has an increased risk of poor health outcomes. For example, being older than age 65 and having a history of hypertension, type 2 diabetes, and atrial fibrillation all increase the client's risk of cardiovascular and neurological diseases. Additionally, the client missing her lisinopril and apixaban medications for the past week increases her risk of elevated blood pressure and of developing clots.

2.

Client Findings	Seizure	Stroke	Hypoglycemia
Aphasia	■	■	■
Gaze deviation	■	■	☐
Unilateral loss of sensation	☐	■	☐
Inability to follow commands	■	■	■
Facial droop	☐	■	☐

Seizures and strokes are both neurological in origin and therefore have overlapping signs and symptoms, including aphasia, gaze deviation, and the inability to follow commands. A stroke is differentiated from a seizure in that the infarct in the brain often results in unilateral deficits, including a unilateral loss of sensation or a facial droop. Hypoglycemia can cause mental status changes, such as the inability to follow commands and even aphasia, but it does not cause unilateral deficits or gaze deviation.

3. 1: The client is most likely experiencing an ischemic stroke based on her symptoms and her recent medical history. Clients with a history of atrial fibrillation who are off of their blood thinning medication are at a higher risk of developing an embolism that could travel to the brain and cause ischemia. The client's symptoms also indicate that she is vision, aphasia, neglect (VAN) positive. This assessment is conducted by a neurologist to determine if the client is likely having a large vessel occlusion. Although diabetes puts the client at a greater risk for strokes, it is unlikely to be considered a direct cause of the stroke. A hemorrhagic stroke is also possible and should be ruled out as soon as possible. However, a hemorrhagic stroke is less likely in this case because the client has not complained of a severe headache and has not had any reported head trauma (such as a fall). Also, missing a dose of a blood thinner such as apixaban is unlikely to cause hemorrhage and more likely to lead to an embolism.

4.

- Obtain serum blood sugar.
- Collect blood for a CBC, BMP, and troponin level.
- Obtain an EKG.
- Provide education on medication compliance.
- Obtain a CT scan of the head.
- Administer IV labetalol.

When dealing with a suspected stroke, it is important to remember that the longer that care is delayed, the more likely the client is to have worse outcomes. Treating a stroke quickly increases the odds that the client will either recover, or at the very least not have worsening symptoms from lack of brain perfusion. Generally, thrombolytics must be administered within 4 hours of the onset of stroke symptoms, and endovascular thrombectomy for large vessel occlusions must be done within 24 hours of the onset of symptoms. A computed tomography (CT) scan of the client should be obtained within 25 minutes of arrival to the emergency department to rule out a hemorrhagic stroke. If indicated, as soon as a hemorrhagic stroke is ruled out (and an ischemic stroke is diagnosed), thrombolytic medication may be administered. Additionally, the client's elevated blood pressure must be treated because a systolic blood pressure above 185 is considered a contraindication for thrombolytics. While it is important to obtain a bedside blood sugar early because hypo-/hyperglycemia can present similarly to a stroke, this was already taken via fingerstick and did not have a concerning finding. Secondary testing such as an electrocardiogram (EKG) and lab work may be done, but this is not a priority and should not delay the initial CT scan or the administration of thrombolytics. Providing patient education about the importance of medication compliance may be important later in the client's care, but it would not be appropriate for the current emergency situation.

5.

Potential Nursing Interventions	Indicated	Not Indicated
Regularly reassess the client's neurological symptoms.	●	○
Request an order for oral lisinopril.	○	●
Regularly recheck the client's vital signs.	●	○
Monitor for signs of facial swelling.	●	○
Request an order for physical therapy.	○	●

When administering thrombolytics, it is important to monitor the client's vital signs and neurological status closely and routinely. Although it is important to note any improvements that the medication may cause, it is also important to quickly recognize and treat any worsening symptoms. Thrombolytics increase the client's risk of hemorrhage, including intracranial hemorrhage. Having an elevated blood pressure can also increase this risk. Additionally, thrombolytics can cause angioedema, which causes facial swelling, that should be recognized and treated early. Although blood pressure medications may be indicated for this client, the client should remain on a strict nothing-by-mouth status until a swallow screening has been completed and shows that she is not at risk of aspiration. Physical therapy will likely be indicated following the client's hospital admission for rehabilitation because she is currently unable to move the right side of her body and would be at a high risk of falling during a physical therapy assessment at this time.

6.

Assessment Findings	Improved	Unchanged	Worsened
Blood pressure, 190/85	○	○	●
Pulse oximetry reading, 92%	○	●	○
NIHSS score, 14	●	○	○
Facial droop	○	●	○
Gaze deviation	●	○	○

The client's overall respiratory assessment has remained unchanged throughout her stay, with the pulse oximetry reading hovering between 92 and 93%. These minor changes remain at suboptimal levels, as a normal pulse oximetry reading is >95% (except for those with conditions such as COPD which is not indicated here). The physician should be notified, as oxygen delivery via nasal cannula may be initiated to increase her oxygenation status to normal range. Her tachypnea (demonstrated by a respiratory rate of >20 breaths per minute) may also improve with oxygen support. The client's overall neurological assessment has improved. The client still seems to have gaze deviation and possible neglect on one side, but she is now able to look to the other side when prompted. Her NIHSS score went from 22 to 14, which is also an improvement (the closer the score is to 0, the better). Her facial droop and most of her vital signs (including her pulse oximetry reading) remain unchanged. However, her blood pressure has worsened. The physician should be notified of this finding immediately. Although the thrombolytic medication was administered nearly 1 hour prior to this, the client is still at risk of intracranial hemorrhage, and her blood pressure needs to be controlled to help prevent that outcome.

Case Study 3

1. 3, 4, and 6: The client's temperature is elevated, which, along with the other symptoms described, is a possible sign of infection. In pediatric clients especially, it is important to monitor for signs of dehydration, which can be caused by diarrhea and vomiting. The client's altered mentation is also concerning because it could be a sign of a disease process such as dehydration or infection, or it could be representative of a postictal state. The client's heart rate, blood pressure, and respiratory rate are within normal limits for his age. The client's pulmonary assessment findings are currently expected. However, the nurse should continue to monitor this closely because his nasal drainage could become an airway blockage, and his mother had reported signs of cyanosis (blue lips) prior to their arrival.

2.

Client Findings	Influenza	UTI	Gastroenteritis
Fever	■	■	■
Cough	■	☐	☐
Diarrhea	☐	☐	■
Loss of appetite	☐	☐	■
Rhinorrhea	■	☐	☐

Influenza, urinary tract infections (UTIs), and gastroenteritis are all infectious disease processes that manifest differently due to the location in which the causative infectious organism colonizes. Influenza virus most often colonizes in the respiratory tract, leading to cough, rhinorrhea, and a fever. That said, influenza in the pediatric population can also cause nausea, vomiting, and diarrhea with a loss of appetite. UTIs are caused by bacterial infection of the urinary tract, leading to a fever, pain on urination, frequent urination, and/or blood in the urine. Gastroenteritis can be caused by viral, bacterial, or parasitic infection in the gastrointestinal tract and results in diarrhea and/or vomiting, abdominal pain, and loss of appetite. In children, gastroenteritis may also cause a fever.

3. 1: Based on the mother's description of the event and the client's presentation (having a high fever and a recent illness), the child most likely experienced a febrile seizure. Because his symptoms have largely resolved upon arrival to the hospital, it is unlikely that he is having an allergic reaction or an asthma exacerbation. Although the mother's description of the event did sound like seizure-like activity, given the client's lack of other medical history and the presence of a fever, it is much less likely that the client had an epileptic event. Febrile seizures are fairly common in young children and generally resolve with age. Should the child continue to have seizures without the presence of a fever or once the child has grown up, further testing may be done to evaluate for the possibility of epilepsy. If he continued to have symptoms such as rash, worsening mentation, or difficulty breathing, these may be possible differential diagnoses to consider.

4.

- Obtain a urinalysis.
- Administer oral acetaminophen suspension.
- Administer oral ondansetron.

- Obtain a stool sample.
- Encourage fluids as tolerated.

The current priority for this client (other than first establishing safety and ensuring that the airway, breathing, and circulation are intact) is to treat his current symptoms in order to prevent a possible repeat seizure and to decrease his chances of dehydration and electrolyte imbalance. The acetaminophen is meant to decrease his fever. The ondansetron is meant to decrease any nausea and vomiting, which will allow him to take in fluids as tolerated and subsequently decrease his dehydration. If the interventions are unsuccessful and the child is unable to tolerate oral fluids, the physician should be notified right away. It is likely that the physician will want to reassess the client. They may want to order more testing (i.e., labs and imaging) and provide IV fluids to maintain the client's electrolytes until symptoms have resolved. Obtaining urine and stool samples may be helpful in diagnosing the cause of his symptoms, but this is not the priority.

5.

Potential Nursing Interventions	Indicated	Not Indicated
Add safety padding to the sides of the client's bed.	●	○
Request that the acetaminophen order be changed to a rectal suppository.	○	●
Request an order for a 1,000 mL IV fluid bolus.	○	●
Provide the client with juice or a Popsicle.	●	○
Provide the client with a cold compress for his forehead/neck.	●	○

Adding safety padding to the sides of the client's bed can reduce the chances of injury if he has another seizure while in the hospital and would be considered a standard seizure precaution. If the client can tolerate oral fluids and the physician does not anticipate any procedures that require sedation, it is important to provide the client with a beverage, broth, or Popsicle to help him replenish his fluid and electrolytes. The cool liquid may also be soothing to his fever. Providing a cold compress may also help lower the client's core body temperature and help control his fever. If the client could not tolerate oral acetaminophen or was too young to take it safely, a rectal suppository may be indicated. However, this client has had diarrhea, which is generally a contraindication for rectal suppository administration. If IV fluid was indicated (i.e., if the client cannot take in enough orally or if his condition worsens), the standard fluid bolus dosage for the pediatric population is 20 mL/kg over 20–30 minutes. Based on the client's weight, 1,000 mL IV fluid would be far more than is indicated (220 mL) and would likely be dangerous to administer. Although the pediatric client can become dehydrated much faster than an adult, he can also become fluid overloaded much quicker. Therefore, it is very important to verify the pediatric client's weight and dosage before administering IV fluids.

6. 2, 3, and 5: Rectally is the most accurate location to measure a child's temperature; the client's mother should be taught how to use this method. If taking a rectal temperature measurement is not possible, the mother should also know how to measure the temporal, tympanic, and axillary temperatures. An oral temperature measurement may be difficult to perform with a child this age because he may not be able to follow directions. Acetaminophen and ibuprofen can help control the child's temperature and decrease discomfort while his body works to fight the disease process. Controlling the child's temperature may also decrease his risk of having another febrile seizure. It is important that parents are educated on the signs and symptoms of dehydration in their children. The mother is incorrect in stating that febrile seizures are the same as an epilepsy diagnosis. The mother should monitor for future seizures, especially those unrelated to fevers. However, it is fairly common for children to have febrile seizures and grow up to never have a seizure again. It is incorrect that the mother should put something in the child's mouth if he has another seizure. This can be dangerous to the mother and to the seizing client. The mother should be educated on how to maintain a safe environment for the child while a seizure is happening, to make note of when the seizure starts and when it ends, record any behaviors the child may have after the seizure, how to monitor for signs of airway obstruction in the child, and when to call for medical help.

Standalone Questions

1. 2: First-degree heart block occurs when the electrical impulse generated by the SA node remains uninterrupted but is delayed through the AV node. First-degree heart block is usually benign. Characteristics of first-degree heart block include a P wave present for every QRS complex, a PR interval of greater than 0.20 s, and no missing beats. If the PR interval extends to more than 0.30 s, the P wave may be hidden in the previous T wave and patients may begin to experience symptoms.

2. 2: If the nurse observes a coworker improperly handling the dispersal of medication, either deliberately or accidentally, the nurse should immediately report the observation to a supervisor. The nurse should not confront the coworker directly as this may result in a verbal conflict and provide warning that the coworker will be investigated.

3. 1, 3, 5, 6: Cold applications block peripheral nerve conduction and provide local anesthesia, so cold may be used to reduce pain. Cold increases the viscosity of the blood, promoting coagulation at a site of injury. Cold also results in vasoconstriction, which reduces edema and inflammation; decreased muscle tension, which helps to prevent muscle spasms; and reduced cell metabolism. Heat applications tend to have the opposite effect, resulting in vasodilation, decreased viscosity of the blood, increased permeability of capillaries, and increased tissue metabolism.

4. Metric weight measures

Milligram	Centigram	Decigram	Gram	Dekagram	Hectogram	Kilogram

1. II
2. I
3. III
4. IV

5. 4: If a mother is concerned that her neonate is having periods of apnea, the nurse should reassure her that slight pauses in breathing, referred to as periodic breathing, are normal in the neonate. Usually the pause is only 2–3 seconds, but it may be longer in some cases. However, if the periods persist for more than 15–20 seconds or increase in frequency, the mother should notify the physician, especially if the episodes are accompanied by other changes, such as pallor, cyanosis, bradycardia, or hypotonia.

6. 1: In this situation, the nurse should remove the ring and secure it according to hospital policy. Most facilities have a secure safe or another area to store valuables until other arrangements can be made. The ring should not be sent home with a family member or caregiver unless this person has power of attorney, is the parent of a client who is a minor, or is a spouse.

7. 3: Headaches occur in about one-fifth of clients following a lumbar puncture, but the headaches are usually relieved by lying flat and drinking ample fluids. If headaches are severe and persistent, then this usually indicates a hole in the dura mater, and an epidural blood patch may be applied with an autologous blood specimen. The blood is injected in a small amount at the site of the lumbar puncture to create a blood clot that serves as a patch.

8. 4: The best method to properly adjust a walker to the correct height is to have the client stand with their arms dangling at their side and then measure the distance from their wrists to the floor. This is the height to which the walker (at the handles) should be adjusted. Walkers are intended for partial weight-bearing only and are not meant to support a client's full weight.

9. 4: While there is not total agreement about the results of HbA1c tests, generally levels at or above 6.5% are considered diagnostic of diabetes mellitus. Values of 5.7–6.4% are considered pre-diabetic by most authorities. Lower values are within normal limits. Because hemoglobin retains excess blood glucose and red blood cells live about 120 days, the HbA1c test shows the average blood glucose levels over a 3-month period. HbA1c is used to diagnose diabetes and monitor long-term diabetic therapy.

10. 1, 2, 4: If a client with COPD asks why they need to have an arterial blood gas (ABG) test, the nurse should explain that ABGs measure the levels of carbon dioxide, oxygen, and acidity (pH level) in the blood, help to evaluate the effectiveness of treatment, and help to determine the need for supplemental oxygen. ABGs are also carried out to help diagnose and monitor certain disorders, such as metabolic disorders and kidney disease.

11. 4: Gait disturbances:

- Parkinsonian gait: slight flexion of hips and knees, short shuffling steps, trunk leaning forward, and no arm swing
- Ataxic gait: uncoordinated and unsteady, wide-based, staggering, high stepping, flat-footed step
- Geriatric gait: decreased speed and balance, slight flexion of hips and knees, stooped posture, and short or decreased stride length
- Scissors gait: short, slow, stiff steps with thighs crossing while moving forward

12. 2, 4: Pills may be crushed and diluted in 10–15 mL of water to be added to the NG tube feedings. Liquid forms of medications are easiest to add. Extended-release capsules should be opened but NOT crushed before adding to the tube. Enteric-coated tablets should not be crushed or administered per NG tube, soft-gel capsules are not recommended because of a tendency to clog the feeding tube despite being dissolved, and sublingual wafers are not absorbed through the GI tract.

13. 3: This is an example of rationalization because the client is attempting to make excuses for drinking excessively. Clients often try to find logical reasons for their actions and often blame their situations, family members, or friends for their problems. With repression, the client involuntarily blocks the awareness of negative feelings and experiences. Suppression is similar to repression, but the blocking of awareness is voluntary. Denial is a refusal to acknowledge that a problem exists at all.

14. 2: The integrity of the closed system of drainage should be maintained. The correct procedure for collecting a urine specimen from a Foley catheter with a sample port is to first wipe the port with alcohol and allow the alcohol to dry. Next, insert a 10-mL needleless syringe into the port and withdraw the sample.

15. Correct order:

1. V. Raise the head of the bed to 30° with the client in the supine position.
2. III. Place the client's upper arm across her chest and roll her to a side-lying position toward the nurse by pulling and supporting her shoulders and hips.
3. IV. Place one arm under the client's shoulders, supporting her head and neck, and place the other arm over her thighs.
4. II. Pivot the client by moving her legs over the side of the bed and elevating her trunk.
5. I. Support the client until she is stable.

16. 2: While there is value in all of these approaches, the best place to begin to gather information about evidence-based practices is to search medical databases, such as Medline Plus, DynaMed Plus, CINAHL, and Cochrane. These resources can provide up-to-date information that is supported by data, which is critical for evidence-based practice. However, the evidence gathered should be carefully assessed for both internal and external validity, including reviewing the numbers of subjects and credentials of the authors.

17. 2: The tasks that may be delegated to the LPN are the dressing change and insertion of a Foley catheter. Checking routine vital signs, giving enemas, and giving bed baths are all within the scope of practice of CNAs, but facility guidelines may vary.

18. 2: Naegele's rule for estimating the due date of a pregnancy is:

- Date of onset of last menstrual period (LMP) + 9 months + 7 days = estimated due date
- September 6 + 9 months = June 6 + 7 days = June 13

Naegele's rule does not account for differences in menstrual cycles or number of days in the months (using an average of 28 days), but this method accounts for approximately 280 days, the normal duration of pregnancy. Most physicians use a combination of Naegele's rule and an ultrasound during the first trimester to estimate a due date.

19. 1, 2, 3, 4: Guillain-Barré syndrome, diabetes mellitus type 1, rheumatoid arthritis, and Hashimoto thyroiditis are all examples of autoimmune disorders. An autoimmune disorder is one in which the client's immune system attacks body tissue. The autoimmune disorder may be systemic, such as with rheumatoid arthritis, or more localized, such as with Hashimoto thyroiditis. About 80 diseases have been identified as autoimmune disorders. Autoimmune disorders often have periods of remission in which symptoms subside, followed by exacerbation of symptoms.

20. 2: Benzodiazepines are usually avoided in frail older adults because of increased risk of falls associated with common adverse effects of drowsiness, sedation, hypotension, and loss of coordination. Benzodiazepines are frequently prescribed as first-line therapy for relief of anxiety, especially generalized anxiety disorder and panic disorder. Benzodiazepines are also sometimes prescribed for insomnia, although in some cases clients have paradoxical reactions in which the client response is the opposite of that expected.

21. 1: When reviewing dietary restriction with an immunocompromised client following kidney transplantation, the client should be advised to avoid raw bean sprouts because of the chance they may harbor pathogenic organisms. Clients should also be advised to avoid grapefruit and grapefruit juice, which may interfere with some medications, as well as raw or undercooked meats and uncooked dough that contains raw eggs, such as cookie dough. Clients should also be advised to limit or avoid foods from buffets or salad bars, as they may not be properly prepared or may sit for prolonged periods, encouraging the growth of bacteria.

22. 1, 3, 4: The nurse should ask the client to describe the hallucinations because this information is necessary to help the nurse calm the client and to determine if the client or others are at risk because of the hallucinations. The nurse should communicate frequently with the client, helping to keep the client oriented and presenting a model of reality. The nurse should also encourage the client to participate in reality-based activities, such as playing cards or badminton. Using distracting techniques is helpful when intervening for delusions but less successful with hallucinations.

23. 1: If a client has suffered an ischemic stroke in the right hemisphere, the nurse should anticipate that the client has left paralysis and left visual field defect. Language skills usually remain intact, although the client may have some short-term memory loss and difficulty following directions. Clients may also act impulsively and have poor judgement. The client's fine motor skills may be impaired, resulting in difficulty dressing and carrying out tasks that involve the use of tools.

24. 2: The food that has the greatest potential for interaction with drugs is grapefruit (both the fruit and the juice) because it contains furanocoumarins, which block the action of CYP3A4 enzymes that metabolize drugs. This can result in increased levels of the drug in the system. Grapefruit interacts with statins, calcium channel blockers, loratadine, and multiple other drugs. Some other fruits, including oranges, apples, pomelos, and pomegranates, may also interact with drugs.

25. 1, 2, 5: Raynaud's disease, intermittent digital arteriolar vasoconstriction, affects the hands and feet and may, with severe vasoconstriction, result in ulceration or gangrene. Vasoconstriction occurs with exposure to cold or stress and is exacerbated by smoking and some medications, so clients should be advised to quit smoking and avoid beta blockers and birth control pills. Treatment may include vasodilators, calcium channel blockers (nifedipine), and sympathectomy.

26. 1, 3, 5: As clients age, their pulmonary elasticity tends to decrease while their chest-wall rigidity increases, making it more difficult to adequately ventilate. Pharyngeal reflexes, which serve a protective role in preventing choking and aspiration, also decrease. Alveoli become distended, decreasing alveolar surface area, and there is ventilation/perfusion mismatching, impairing the exchange of oxygen. Older adults undergoing surgery may need extended preoxygenation prior to surgery and higher concentrations of oxygen during the procedure to avoid hypoxia.

27. 2: If the client has stress incontinence while playing golf, she should certainly be encouraged to urinate immediately before playing golf and to wear incontinence pads for security, but the most effect technique is likely the "knack," which is the use of precisely timed muscle contractions (Kegel exercises). The client should contract the pelvic muscles immediately before stressful events, such as the golf swing, and maintain the contraction until the event is over. This maneuver provides support to the proximal urethra, preventing incontinence.

28. 1: The initial step that the nurse should take to protect the wound is to cover it with saline-soaked sterile dressings to keep the tissue moist and prevent irritation. Evisceration requires emergent surgical intervention to prevent sepsis. The head of the bed should be elevated to semi-Fowler's position and the knees slightly flexed to reduce tension on the wound.

29. 3: There is no antidote for an overdose of muscle relaxants, such as baclofen. Therefore, treatment consists of supportive care. The client should receive large volumes of intravenous fluids to prevent the development of crystalluria, and they may require mechanical ventilation if respirations are severely depressed. The client should be placed on cardiac monitoring. If other CNS depressant drugs are taken along with the overdose of muscle relaxant, the client is more at risk.

30. 1: The cephalic presentation that is most common during delivery of a neonate is the vertex presentation. With this presentation, the fetal head is fully flexed and the diameter is the smallest,

38. 1, 2, 3, 4: If a client has suffered a traumatic brain injury and is being treated in the ICU, the nurse should expect to elevate the head of the bed and keep the client's head in neutral alignment. The nurse will likely administer oxygen to maintain the SpO2 at >90% (less than this is considered hypoxemia) and will administer sedation to prevent or reduce agitation. Additionally, cerebral perfusion pressure should be maintained between 60-70 mmHg and body temperature should be maintained within normal limits.

39. 4: If a client's medication order is for 300 mg of a liquid medication that is available at 75 mg per mL, the nurse should administer 4 mL of medication.

$$\frac{(300 \text{ mg})}{75 \text{ mg/mL}} = 4 \text{ mL}$$

40. 1, 2, 4, 5: In this situation, the client should receive the 72-hour N-acetylcysteine (NAC) protocol and supportive care in an attempt to minimize hepatic damage. Hepatic function must be monitored carefully. It is too late for GI contamination with activated charcoal. The Rumack-Matthew nomogram is used to determine the need for treatment. The client should also receive a psychiatric consultation.

41. 1: If the nurse is caring for a client in the recovery room after the client's abdominal surgery and the BP is initially stable but then falls 5 or more mmHg every 15 minutes, the nurse should notify the surgeon, as this may be an indication of bleeding and/or the development of shock. Generally, the surgeon should be notified if the systolic BP falls below 90, but the nurse should not wait since a clear pattern of decreasing blood pressure is evident.

42. 4: Decreasing inflammation may reduce edema. Methylprednisolone is a steroidal anti-inflammatory drug used to control spinal cord edema. Mannitol is an osmotic diuretic used to control brain edema. Aspirin and morphine do not affect spinal cord inflammation, as they are analgesics.

43. 1: The nurse should hold the infusion and notify the MD that the catheter tip is incorrectly placed, as it should be in the superior vena cava rather than the right atrium. Infusing the solutions directly into the right atrium may result in tissue damage. While the catheter needs to be withdrawn a few inches and another x-ray taken to ensure correct placement, this procedure should only be done by a physician or a specially trained nurse.

44. 2, 3, 5: If the nurse is examining a client's incision following a radical nephrectomy, signs or symptoms that indicate infection include tissue around the incision being moderately edematous and increasingly erythematous, a foul odor from the wound dressing, and evidence of purulent discharge. Slight serosanguineous discharge is common and usually not cause for concern. Pain in the incisional area in the postoperative period is very common and usually does not indicate infection unless there is a change in the character of the pain and other signs or symptoms are present.

45. 2, 4: If a client has accidentally splashed a toxic (although not caustic) substance in the right eye, the steps to flushing the eye include:

- Place the client on their right side and elevate their head to 20 degrees.
- Hold the emesis basin against the right side of their face.
- Fill bulb syringe with NS irrigant.
- Hold the right eyelid open with the thumb and index finger.

- Hold the tip of the syringe about a half-inch above the eye and direct the flow of the irrigant toward the lower conjunctival sac, from inner to outer canthus.
- Flush for about 1 minute.

46. 2: The wound shows evidence of erythema and edema, and phagocytosis begins during the inflammation stage of injury repair. Stages:

1. Hemostasis: During first few minutes. Platelets seal off the vessels and secrete substances that cause vasoconstriction. Thrombin stimulates the clotting mechanism, forming a fibrin mesh.
2. Inflammation: Over days 1–4. Inflammatory response and phagocytosis occur.
3. Proliferation: Over days 5–20. Fibroblasts produce collagen and granulation tissue starts to form. Epithelialization contracts wound.
4. Maturation: After day 21 to 2 years. Collagen tightens to reduce scarring. The tissue gains tensile strength.

47. 1, 2, 3: The long-term effects of prolonged use of phenytoin include a condition referred to as "Dilantin facies," which is characterized by gingival hypertrophy, hirsutism, and hypertrophy of facial subcutaneous tissue. Clients must be advised to maintain good dental care. Additionally, clients may develop osteoporosis, so supplementary vitamin D is usually advised. Clients with low levels of albumin (usually associated with renal disease or malnutrition) may have more severe effects.

48. 2: The client is probably in the anger stage of the grief process (Kübler-Ross). Upon receiving bad news, many clients initially experience **denial**, although this period usually only lasts one to two weeks. Within a few hours of receiving bad news, many also begin to experience **anger**, and this anger is often directed at family members and caregivers because clients feel helpless and terrified. Many also go through a **bargaining** stage where they may begin attending religious services or seek other opinions. **Depression** may be prolonged as the client comes to grips with loss and finally reaches **acceptance**.

49. 1: Clients taking anticholinergic drugs to relieve muscle tremors and muscle rigidity associated with Parkinson disease should be advised to avoid overheating. Clients taking anticholinergics should be advised to avoid high environmental temperatures or activities, which may increase internal temperature, such as excessive exercise during warm weather. Because anticholinergics interfere with the body's ability to perspire, the body cannot adequately cool if overheated. Anticholinergics are often used as adjuncts to primary Parkinson drugs.

50. 2, 3: Positive reinforcement provides something in return for a change in behavior. This can include tangible rewards, such as an additional hour of Internet use or some type of privilege, or supportive statements, such as "You are making good progress." When possible, positive reinforcement should occur immediately after a behavioral change so that the client makes a positive association with the behavior.

51. 4: If, when inserting a nasogastric feeding tube, the nurse pauses after inserting the tube 25 cm, this is at the level of the carina. If the nurse listens at the distal end of the tube and hears air exchange, this is an indication that the tube is in the respiratory tract and not the esophagus. The tube should be immediately completely withdrawn, allowing the client time to relax and stop coughing, before insertion is attempted again. Note, even if there is no sound of air exchange, this cannot be used as confirmation of correct placement.

52. 30: The problem can be calculated using dimensional analysis:

$$\frac{120 \text{ mL}}{1 \text{ hour}} \times \frac{15 \text{ drops}}{1 \text{ mL}} \times \frac{1 \text{ hour}}{60 \text{ min}}$$

Eliminate like terms (mL and hour) and reduce 120/60:

$$\frac{2}{1} \times \frac{15 \text{ drops}}{1} \times \frac{1}{1 \text{ min}} = 30 \frac{\text{drops}}{\text{min}}$$

53. 2: If a physician has telephoned a number of orders for a client who has developed a fever and chills, the nurse should write the orders in their entirety and then read them back to confirm that the orders are correct. However, if an order is not clear, then the nurse should clarify that order when it is given. The nurse may repeat the individual orders while writing them, but should not routinely stop with each order to confirm, as this interrupts the physician's flow of thought and may be distracting.

54. 1, 2: Disguising the doorway by hanging a curtain across it or placing a painting on the door is enough to prevent some clients with dementia from opening the door. A good way to keep clients inside is to place a latch at the top or bottom of the door, as Alzheimer's clients rarely look beyond the doorknob when trying to open a door. Clients should never be locked into a room, and motion sensors with alarms are often terrifying to clients, increasing their stress and need to get away.

55. 3: If the nurse notes that a transfer procedure is time consuming because of redundant steps and has develop a streamlined procedure, the nurse should propose the new procedure to the performance improvement committee so that the procedure can be reviewed and a decision made about implementation. Once procedures have been established, questioning them and revising those that are inefficient are important steps, but these should not be carried out unilaterally.

56. 3: The most helpful information for the homeless client is probably a list of shelters and community agencies, especially those with programs to assist the homeless. Adult Protective Services investigates abuse, but cuts resulting from a fight are not usually considered abusive situations. Many homeless people are very reluctant to deal with the police in any way. Providing a list of 12-step organizations is not indicated unless the client is inebriated or there is other evidence of a drinking problem.

57. 4: Skeletal muscle tremor can show up as an electrical artifact on ECG tracings. It classically looks like irregular, spiky oscillations of the baseline, and may mimic atrial fibrillation or other cardiac abnormalities. It is necessary to determine the cause of the tremor and to find a way to prevent recurring tremors during the ECG. If the patient is tense, provide reassurance and ask them to relax. If they are cold, ensure the room is warm and provide blankets. If they have Parkinson's disease or another cause of tremor, move the limb electrodes closer to the torso or have the patient tuck their hands under their body.

58. 1, 3, 4, 5: Energy-conservation techniques include sitting down to perform activities instead of standing. The client should keep frequently used items close at hand but at arm level, so the person does not have to reach up or bend down because these activities require increased energy. The client should plan ahead to avoid extra movements; ask for help when needed; and use correct body mechanics, including pushing items instead of pulling them. The client should be advised to watch for stress signals, such as dyspnea or fatigue.

59. 1: In this situation, the best response is to provide supportive care as indicated and respect the client's right to refuse treatment. While it is appropriate to tell the client that he can change his mind at any time, pressuring the client or his family is not appropriate.

60. 1, 3, 4, 5: In this situation, the nurse should advise the client to take the medication at bedtime because it may cause the client to become sedated or to develop postural hypotension. Additionally, the client may need to take a stool softener because the drug may cause dry mouth and constipation. The client should be advised to report urinary or sexual dysfunction, common adverse effects.

61. 3: A Glasgow Coma Scale (GCS) score of 6 indicates a coma. GCS is based on scores assigned for three parameters: eye-opening response, verbal response, and muscle response. Scores range from 3 (worst possible) to 15 (best possible). Head injuries are classified according to the following scores:

- Coma: GCS score of 3–8
- Severe head injury: GCS score of 8 or less
- Moderate head injury: GCS score of 9–12
- Mild head injury: GCS score of 13–15

62. 1, 2, 3, 6: If a client has recurrent episodes of constipation and fecal impaction, interventions that should be part of bowel training include scheduled toileting, such as attempting to defecate at the same time each day. The client should be advised to increase fluid intake and eat high-fiber foods. Stool softeners may be taken but not daily laxatives, which may in time make constipation worse. Stimulants, such as a suppository or a hot cup of coffee, may help to promote defecation. Routine exercise may help to stimulate intestinal contractions.

63. 1: If a nurse must move a heavy cart full of supplies, the technique that uses the best body mechanics is to push the cart from behind with both hands, keeping the head up, back straight, and knees bent to prevent muscle injury. The nurse should avoid pulling or twisting when moving items and should stand close to the item that is being pushed rather than standing at a distance and leaning into it.

64. 3: In this situation, the nurse should immediately block the view or close-out the screen to prevent the coworker from reading, as this is a breach of confidentiality. Only those who are authorized to access a client's record may legally do so. If a nurse allows others to view the record, this nurse is also at fault.

65. 1: In this situation, the immediate response before notifying the physician should be to clamp the catheter and place the client in left lateral Trendelenburg position to prevent the air from entering the right side of the heart and the pulmonary arteries. These signs and symptoms are indicative of an air embolism. The client may be provided oxygen as necessary.

66. 1, 2, 4: Clients with a tracheostomy are at increased risk of fecal impaction because they cannot perform the Valsalva maneuver to bear down, so they need to be educated about bowel care and advised to use stool softeners routinely and laxatives and suppositories as needed. Additionally, they need to understand the importance of pulmonary hygiene to prevent atelectasis and infection and should be confident in all aspects of tracheostomy care, including information about what to do if the tracheostomy tube falls out.

67. 2: This ECG tracing is typical of left bundle branch block. The QRS duration is ≥0.12 s. The QRS complex is widened because activation of the left ventricle is delayed.

- Lead V1: The QRS complex is negative, with a "W" appearance and a dominant S wave. The R wave may be small, or there may be no preceding R wave.
- Lead V6: The QRS complex is broad and positive. The R wave is broad, with a notched "M" appearance.

68. 4: In this situation, the initial intervention should be to assess the client's cardiac and respiratory status before deciding how to proceed. The nurse should never assume to know the reason for a client's symptoms without conducting an assessment.

69. 2: In this situation, the nurse is at risk of developing varicella zoster virus (chickenpox) if not previously vaccinated. Shingles results from reactivation of the varicella zoster virus, so in order to develop shingles, the individual must first be infected with chickenpox. Once the blisters of shingles have crusted over, the client is no longer contagious.

70. 1: If a nurse believes that current procedures should be changed, then the best place to begin is with a survey of the literature regarding wound care to determine what best practices are recommended. Armed with this information, the nurse can approach the director of nursing or another appropriate person and discuss other methods, such as interviews and questionnaires, which might help to determine the need for change, those interested in assisting, and the best way to proceed.

71. The correct order for the clean intermittent catheterization (CIC) procedure is as follows:

6. (Step 1) III. Spread labia and cleanse area with soap and water.
7. (Step 2) I. Locate meatus (by touch or by using a mirror).
8. (Step 3) IV. Lubricate catheter (with water-soluble lubricant)
9. (Step 4) II. Insert catheter and hold in place until urine stops draining.

The catheter is then removed and discarded if disposable or cleaned according to manufacturer's directions for future use.

72. 4: Because the client is nulliparous, the average rate of dilation is 1 cm per hour, so the approximate time to full dilation of 10 cm is approximately 7 hours. The woman has been progressing at the average rate. The latent phase of stage 1 usually lasts 10–14 hours, and the client was in this phase for 12 hours and has now progressed to the active phase. However, the nurse should stress to the client that there are individual variations with some progressing much more quickly and others more slowly.

73. 3: In this situation, the nurse should immediately begin to make a list of noncritical clients who might be safely discharged so that discharge plans can be made quickly if the need arises. The nurse should avoid calling physicians and tying up the phone lines until receiving more specific information.

facilitating passage through the birth canal. In most cases, the fetal attitude (relationship of body parts to each other) is flexion and the lie (relationship of fetal long axis to mother's) is longitudinal. Complications may arise if the presentation, lie, and/or attitude are different.

31. 1,080: Calculation:

$$8 + 4 + 6 + 4 + 8 + 6 = 36$$
$$(36 \text{ oz}) \times \frac{30 \text{ mL}}{1 \text{ oz}} = 1,080 \text{ mL}$$

Note that ice cream and gelatin dessert are considered as liquids when calculating intake and output.

32. 3: Although brain damage can occur during labor and delivery, it is more often caused by a lack of oxygen than from compression. In most cases, compression results in cranial molding, which is a relatively benign condition that resolves within a few days of birth. Compression occurs during the second stage of labor, with molding being more pronounced if there is a disparity between the size of the fetal head and the maternal bony pelvis. The bones of the baby's skull are soft and flexible with sutures that allow the plates of the skull to overlap if necessary.

33. 3: Physical signs and symptoms of menopause include increased fat deposits on the hips and abdomen, often associated with weight gain and decreased metabolic rate. Clients may have difficulty sleeping and develop restless leg syndrome and heart palpitations. Hot flashes are common. Clients lose subcutaneous fat in the labia and are more at risk for problems with the lower urinary tract, such as stress incontinence and bladder and vaginal infections.

34. 3: Without being overly technical or overly simplistic ("sound . . . was normal"), the nurse should explain to the daughter that trapped air escaped from the lungs when the client was moved. The nurse should also explain other changes to expect, such as a cooling of the body temperature (1.0–1.8 °C/hour) and discoloring of dependent tissues (liver mortis). In most cases, the client's body is transported to a funeral home prior to the onset of rigor mortis (2–4 hours), but the daughter should be advised of this also if the wait time is longer.

35. 1: Incidental teaching uses a child's interests as teaching opportunities and motivation to respond for those with autism spectrum disorder. This type of teaching is not classroom-based. The best example is when the nurse asks, "What color is the bunny?" and waits for a correct response before giving the child the desired toy. Questions should be appropriate for the child's age and abilities. Objective questions are easier for children with autism spectrum disorder than subjective questions.

36. 2: Failure to sense may result in either over- or undersensing and occurs when the pacemaker is unable to detect intrinsic cardiac activity, resulting in pacing randomly at inappropriate times. The pacing spike, for example, may occur within the QRS complex. If the spike occurs within the T wave, this can result in R-on-T arrhythmias, which can lead to ventricular fibrillation or VT. Failure to sense can be caused by lead displacement, depleted battery, incorrect sensitivity settings, and myocardial infarction.

37. 3: If a client with bipolar disorder is exhibiting disturbed thought processes as evidenced by delusional thinking, the nurse should avoid arguing or challenging the client. Instead, the nurse should indicate acceptance and reasonable doubt: "I understand you believe this, but I don't see evidence that this is true." The nurse should try to refocus the client's thoughts to reality by talking about real events and people rather than allowing the client to continue to focus on the delusion.

74. 675: If a 4-year-old client weighing 39.6 pounds is to receive an infusion of IV ceftriaxone sodium at 75 mg/kg/d in a divided dose every 12 hours, the child should receive 675 mg with each infusion. First, convert the weight in pounds (lb) to kilograms (kg), then multiply the result by the dosage.

$$\frac{39.6 \text{ lb}}{2.2 \text{ lb/kg}} = 18 \text{ kg}$$

$$(75 \text{ mg/kg/day}) \times (18 \text{ kg}) = 1{,}350 \text{ mg/day}$$

The total dose is given in divided doses every 12 hours, and since there are two 12-hour periods in a day:

$$\frac{1{,}350 \text{ mg/day}}{2 \text{ doses/day}} = 675 \text{ mg}$$

75. 4: The fracture that poses the greatest risk to older adults is the hip/femur fracture, most often involving the femoral neck and the intertrochanteric region. During initial treatment, mortality rates are 10% with over 25% dying over the following year. Hip fractures often occur because of weakness in the bones resulting from osteoporosis and, in fact, the fracture may be spontaneous, causing the client to fall rather than the result of a fall.

76. 1, 2, 3, 4: In this situation, the nurse should advise the client of the health risks of leaving before treatment is completed, assess the client's mental status and ability to make decisions, ask the client to sign an AMA form, and arrange for some type of follow-up, such as a phone call or return visit. The client should be provided with necessary discharge information, such as the treatment provided and the plan of care, as well as contact information for the physician or other healthcare providers.

77. 2: Panic attacks usually subside within 5–30 minutes, and the best nursing response is to stay with the client while the panic attack occurs, speaking in a calm reassuring voice even though the client in the acute stage may not be processing verbal input. Maintaining the client's safety is a primary concern because during panic attacks clients may bolt and run, even sometimes injuring themselves in the process. Quieting the environment and reducing stimuli may help reduce the client's anxiety.

78. 1, 3: The client should receive the following instructions on the proper use of the assistive device:

1. The client should always grasp the bar with both hands before moving in order to move smoothly and prevent straining the muscles.
2. After grasping the bar, the client should flex the unaffected (in this case left) knee and hip and place the foot flat on the bed.
3. In one movement, the client should pull on the trapeze while pushing down on the left foot and moving the body.

79. 3: The obstetric history of this client would be classified as gravida 4, para 3. Gravida refers to the number of pregnancies, regardless of the duration or outcome. Para refers to the number of births after 20 weeks, regardless of whether they are live births or not. This client had 4 total pregnancies (gravida 4) and 3 births after 20 weeks (para 3).

80. 2: If at all possible, each treatment should be documented immediately after completion. Treatments should never be documented in advance, even if they are routine and the nurse is relatively sure they will be completed. The longer the period of time following completion of a treatment, the greater the chance that an error in documenting (such as forgetting to chart) will occur. If the nurse cannot document immediately, then the nurse should make a note of the time and essential information. Documenting should not be left until the end of shift.

81. 4: Because naloxone (Narcan) reverses the action of opioids, if administered to a long-time opioid user, it may trigger a severe withdrawal reaction and seizures. The dosage of naloxone should be titrated carefully and the client should be monitored throughout treatment. Withdrawal symptoms may occur within minutes of administration of the drug, depending on the dosage of medication and the degree of opioid dependence.

82. 2: When assessing a client with the timed up and go (TUG) test, the normal time required for a client to complete standing, walking 3 meters, turning, returning back, and sitting down is 7–10 seconds. If the client requires 14 seconds or longer, this indicates increased risk for falls. The nurse may also assess gait speed in 5 meters. If the client walks at a rate slower than 0.6 meters/second, this is predictive of mobility limitations.

83. 1: The sterile field extends from the waist to the shoulders, and sterile gowns are considered sterile only between these points. Any sterile item that is held out of the line of sight or below the waist is considered contaminated. The sterile field should be placed on a table that is waist high. The drape is considered sterile except for one inch around the perimeter of the drape, so no contents should come in contact with that area. Sterile items should be dropped toward the center of the drape.

84. 2: Even though a medication error may seem relatively harmless, any time an error is made, the proper procedures must be followed. These include notifying the client's physician, documenting the actual medication given on the client's record (without indicating that it was given in error), and filing an incident report that describes in detail how the incident occurred. Individual institutions may have specific reporting protocols that must be followed, such as requiring a report to risk management or a supervisor.

85. 1, 2, 4: If a client with heart failure has a left ventricular fraction of 38%, this is classified as heart failure (<40% EF). Normal EF is 50–70%. Risk of dysrhythmias occurs if the EF falls to below 35%. While the client should avoid strenuous exercise and should take frequent rest periods, maintaining a routine of regular exercise, such as walking, is important to maintain adequate cardiac output. The client should stop smoking and limit alcohol intake to one to two drinks daily.

86. 4: The client is probably practicing thought-stopping. This is a technique that people sometimes use to stop the intrusion of negative thoughts or anxiety. Initially, clients learn the technique by imagining something that causes them to have negative thoughts, such as the fear of being in public, and then they shout, "STOP," and attempt to redirect thoughts. Over time, they speak the word "stop" and then may substitute a silent thought. Some people use the snap of a rubber band against the skin to stop thoughts.

87. 3: The dressing type that is most appropriate for a stage II pressure injury with moderate amounts of exudate is the hydrocolloid dressing, which contains gelling agents, which help to absorb exudate. NS and gauze (wet-to-dry) dressings are no longer recommended because they disturb granulating tissue. Transparent film is not appropriate for exudative wounds because it has no absorptive properties. Hydrogel dressings are designed to hydrate dry wounds and are not used for wounds with exudate.

88. 4: If the nurse is planning to empty a Jackson-Pratt drainage device but notes a number of large clots in the tubing, the nurse should milk the tubing to move the clots into the device before emptying it. The nurse may use an alcohol swab to facilitate the process. The nurse begins by pinching off the tubing at the distal end and, using an alcohol swab wrapped around the tubing, squeezing the tubing with fingers of the other hand, and sliding a short distance down the tubing, forcing the clots to move down. This procedure is repeated the length of the tubing.

89. 2: Vitamin B9 (folic acid/folate) is necessary to prevent neural tube defects. These defects of the brain, spinal cord, and/or spine occur within the first month of pregnancy, so women who are planning a pregnancy should begin taking the vitamin prior to becoming pregnant and then continue taking the vitamin throughout pregnancy. Most multivitamins contain folic acid, and it may also be included in enriched cereals. Dietary sources of folate (the naturally occurring form) include dark-green leafy vegetables such as spinach, mustard greens, and collard greens as well as beets, broccoli, lentils, and other beans.

90. 2, 3, 4, 5: The American Medical Association has developed guidelines for informed consent. Components include:

- Explanation of diagnosis
- Nature of, and reason for, treatment or procedure
- Risks and benefits
- Alternative options (regardless of cost or insurance coverage)
- Risks and benefits of alternative options
- Risks and benefits of not having a treatment or procedure

Clients should have a good understanding of the procedure itself and the risks and possible complications associated with a procedure. Clients should not in any way be coerced into signing an informed consent form.

91. 1, 3, 4: Contraindications to levodopa include narrow-angle glaucoma, pregnancy, and melanoma (or suspicious skin lesions that may be melanoma). Additionally, levodopa should not be given to clients with psychoses and must be monitored carefully if administered to clients with a history of cardiac problems. Levodopa interacts with numerous drugs, so the client's list of medications should be reviewed by a pharmacist.

92. 1, 2, 3: Normalization is the process of providing a child with as normal an environment as possible in a facility, such as a hospital. Rooms may be painted in bright colors and play areas may be provided. Visiting hours are usually unrestricted, and siblings (and sometimes therapy animals) are allowed to visit. Children may eat in communal areas and be allowed more choices related to foods and sleeping hours. Planned play activities and group activities may be available for children as well. Doll reenactment is a therapeutic play technique.

93. 3: If a client who has never received a measles vaccination was exposed to a child with measles 14 days earlier, the client is at risk for another 7 days as the incubation period ranges from 7–21 days (average onset is at 14 days). Additionally, if the client is infected, she can pass the disease to others from 4 days prior to onset of rash to 4 days after. Measles is an airborne disease that is spread by body fluids. If an infected person coughs and spreads the virus, the virus can remain airborne for an hour.

94. 2: Brain tumors or traumatic brain injuries to different parts of the brain can result in specific types of symptoms:

- Frontal lobe: Changes in mood and personality, as well as hemiparesis
- Occipital lobe: Visual disturbances and visual hallucinations
- Temporal lobe: Loss of memory, speech abnormalities, and lack of coordination
- Parietal lobe: Loss of sensation; difficulty with fine motor skills, such as writing; and loss of half-body awareness
- Cerebellum: Lack of balance and coordination
- Brain stem: Dysphagia, facial pain, weakness, and cranial nerve dysfunction

95. 250: Calculation:

$$\left(\frac{15\ \text{drops}}{1\ \text{min}}\right) \times \left(\frac{1\ \text{ml}}{15\ \text{drops}}\right) = 1\ \text{ml/min}$$

$$(250\ \text{ml}) \times (1\ \text{ml/min}) = 250\ \text{min}$$

96. 3: This type of lesion would be classified as a macule. Macular lesions include those associated with petechiae, measles, and scarlet fever. Freckles are benign macules. A patch is similar to a macule but larger than 1 cm. Papules are solid, elevated, and less than 1 cm in diameter. Nodules are similar to papules but larger than 1 cm.

97. 4: This ECG recording represents premature ventricular contraction (PVC). PVCs are ectopic beats that can occur early in otherwise healthy individuals, although they are of concern in those with preexisting heart disease because they may indicate a risk for more severe ventricular arrhythmias, such as ventricular tachycardia. The impulse for the ectopic beat originates within the ventricles prior to the sinus impulse. PVCs may occur singly, in pairs, or in a recurring pattern and are often followed by a compensatory pause.

98. 2: Temperatures for hot and cold applications:

- Hot: 37–41 °C (98–106 °F)
- Warm: 34–37 °C (93–98 °F)
- Lukewarm: 26–34 °C (80–93 °F)
- Cool: 18–26 °C (65–80 °F)
- Cold: 10–18 °C (50–65 °F)

Hot and cold applications should be limited to durations of 10–20 minutes because longer periods may result in tissue damage. Because moisture conducts heat, hot compresses increase the risk of burns.

99. 1: In this situation, the nurse should ask the parents for advice about managing the child's behavior because comfort measures may be very individual with autism. If possible, at least one parent should remain with the child at all times.

100. 2: The pH in this situation usually indicates intestinal aspirate rather than gastric aspirate. Gastric aspirate may vary in color from cloudy to green to tan to brown with a pH less than 4, while intestinal aspirate may be yellow or brown but the pH is usually greater than 4. Respiratory secretions may look like saliva and have a pH greater than 5.5.

www.ingramcontent.com/pod-product-compliance
Lightning Source LLC
Chambersburg PA
CBHW061325190326
41458CB00011B/3899

* 9 7 8 1 5 1 6 7 0 8 1 1 6 *